All You Really Need To Know To Interpret Arterial Blood Gases

All You Really Need To Know To Interpret Arterial Blood Gases

LAWRENCE MARTIN, M.D., FACP, FCCP
Chief, Division of Pulmonary and Critical Care Medicine
Mt. Sinai Medical Center, Cleveland

Associate Professor of Medicine
Case Western Reserve University School of Medicine

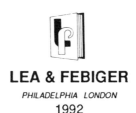

LEA & FEBIGER
PHILADELPHIA LONDON
1992

Lea & Febiger
200 Chester Field Parkway
Malvern, Pennsylvania 19355-9725
U.S.A.
(215) 251-2230

Library of Congress Cataloging-in-Publication Data

Martin, Lawrence, 1943-
  All you really need to know to interpret arterial blood gases / Lawrence Martin.
    p.   cm.
  Includes bibliographical references and index.
  ISBN 0-8121-1572-4
  1. Blood gases — Analysis. I. Title.
  [DNLM: 1. Blood Gas Analysis — methods — programmed instruction. QY 18
  M381a]
  RB45.M37   1992
  616.07'561 — dc20
  DNLM/DLC
  for Library of Congress   92-6255
                                                                           CIP

DISCLAIMER: This book is about how to interpret arterial blood gas data in the clinical setting. Although many patient examples are included, no book, including this one, can tell what to do in a specific clinical situation. Depending on the clinical setting identical blood gas results can lead to very different clinical strategies. The author accepts no responsibility for any action or inaction on the part of any individual that may be based on information in this book.

Reprints of chapters may be purchased from Lea & Febiger in quantities of 100 or more. Contact Sally Grande in the Sales Department.

PRINTED IN THE UNITED STATES OF AMERICA

Print number: 5   4

DEDICATION

To the medical students of Case Western Reserve University
and to the Department of Medicine housestaff, Mt. Sinai
Medical Center, Cleveland

Preface: A Basic Test

There are a few basic tests used in the care of patients. A basic test is one that is applicable to a broad group of patients, provides invaluable information quickly, can be repeated as often as necessary, and is not dependent on patient effort for accuracy. My short list of such essential tests (in alphabetical order):

1. arterial blood gases
2. chest x-ray
3. complete blood count (CBC)
4. electrocardiogram
5. Gram's stain for bacteria
6. serum electrolytes, BUN and glucose
7. urine analysis.

No doubt, the better we understand information provided by these few tests, the better we can care for our patients. CT scans, echocardiograms, perfusion scans, Doppler studies, enzyme assays, spirometry, and other tests of specific organ function (e.g., thyroid, liver, pancreas) certainly have their place, and are at times crucial to diagnosis. However the seven tests listed above, along with the medical history and physical examination, form a foundation for managing virtually all inpatients and a great many chronically ill outpatients.

The newest test on this list to become routinely available is arterial blood gases. The first arterial puncture was performed in 1912 by Hurter, a German physician. In 1919 arterial blood gas analysis was first used as a diagnostic procedure. Employing Hurter's radial artery puncture technique, W.C. Stadie measured oxygen saturation in patients with pneumonia and showed that cyanosis of critically ill patients resulted from incomplete oxygenation of hemoglobin (Stadie 1919).

Over the next 40 years blood gas measurements were more of a laboratory research tool than a test available for everyday patient care. Techniques for measuring blood gases required specialized apparatus and were difficult to perform. It was not until the 1950s that electrodes were developed that could rapidly and reproducibly measure PaO_2, $PaCO_2$ and pH.

Preface (continued)

In 1953 Leland Clark invented the platinum oxygen electrode, a prototype that evolved into the first modern blood gas electrode (Clark 1953, Clark 1956). Development of commercially viable pH and PCO_2 electrodes soon followed and by the mid-1960s several university centers were able to provide pH, $PaCO_2$ and PaO_2 measurements on arterial blood, albeit using cumbersome and non-automated equipment. In 1973 the first commercially available, automated blood gas machine was introduced (ABL1 from Radiometer), and this was soon followed by machines from other companies (Severinghaus 1986). Today virtually every acute care hospital provides rapid and automated blood gas testing 24 hours a day, 7 days a week.

As performed by electrodes on a single sample of arterial blood, the ABG test now has competition: non-invasive measurements. Particularly popular, and replacing the need for some arterial sample-based tests, are pulse oximeters for measuring oxygen saturation and end-tidal gas analysis for PCO_2. In neonates and small children, skin electrodes for measuring PO_2 and PCO_2 have found wide application.

Even more exciting is the new technology for measuring blood gases *continuously*, using tiny fiberoptic sensors that fit inside the blood vessel. Although an invasive technique, optical sensing promises to add a new dimension to monitoring changes in pH, $PaCO_2$ and PaO_2.

Whatever the technology, the important thing is the information and its proper clinical application. All blood gas technologies are designed to provide information on oxygenation, ventilation and/or acid-base balance through one or more measurements. Teaching you how to interpret and wisely use blood gas values — no matter how they are obtained — is the goal of this book.

This is not a physiology textbook. I have left out some aspects of blood gas physiology that, while interesting, are not crucial to learning basic blood gas interpretation; examples include the shunt equation, the carbon dioxide dissociation curve, and the Fick equation for oxygen uptake. Nor is this a compendium of all clinical situations. Omitted are discussions of blood gases during

Preface (continued)

the neonatal period, mixed venous oxygen measurements, and blood gas alterations during hyperbaric therapy. The bibliography provides several references where one can find discussion of these and other specialized topics.

Rather than produce an encyclopedia that covers everything lightly, I have tried to create a work that will, first and foremost, teach the important aspects in depth and be clinically useful. The vast majority of people who use arterial blood gases in the care of patients should find in this book all they "really need to know."

Lawrence Martin, M.D.

ACKNOWLEDGMENTS

Along the way many students and physicians reviewed portions of this work. Their comments and criticisms, always appreciated, have helped me to refine the book and keep its focus on *clinical practice*. Special acknowledgment goes to Ian Cohen, M.D. for his careful review of the entire manuscript. I also want to thank artist Debra Shirley and the staff of Mt. Sinai Hospital's Visual Media Shop for their valuable assistance. Finally, I particularly want to thank Mr. Brian Jeffreys, who runs our blood gas lab, for his continued support and collaboration on our many "projects."

Table of Contents

(continued)

Table of Contents (continued)

How to Use This Book for Maximum Benefit

1. Get a pencil.

   This is a very practical book about an important laboratory test, arterial blood gases. The book's emphasis is on interpreting blood gases in the clinical setting. Real patients and real clinical situations are presented along the way.

   Don't read this book without a pencil in hand. You won't need a calculator and paper is optional; the necessary arithmetic can be done in the book itself. But go get a pencil. Without applying pencil to paper — answering the multiple-choice questions and doing some simple calculations before checking your answers — you won't be forced to think about the problems presented. And you won't get the maximum value out of the book.

   Answers to the numbered questions (e.g., 2-1, 2-2) are at the end of each chapter. Questions without numbers are answered in the paragraphs immediately following; they are signified by a ? just before the list of possible answers.

   QUESTIONS:
   Numbered: Answered at end of chapter
   Not numbered: Answered in subsequent
   paragraphs

   You should answer *all* questions with a pencil as they are encountered, then check your answers. Follow this advice and you cannot help but learn the fundamentals of blood gas interpretation. If you skip the pencil you won't know whether the information has registered or whether you have really learned what's important. Applying pencil to paper is the only reliable way to *learn* what the book attempts to teach you.

   So go get a pencil.

How to Use This Book for
Maximum Benefit (continued)

2. Take the Pre-test, then check your answers (Appendix B).

3. Read the Introduction to Quik-Course, page xxi. Then, either review the Quik-Course (Chapter 10) or begin with Chapter 1, page 1.

4. Read the chapters at your own pace, always stopping to answer each question *with your pencil.*

5. Make sure you understand all the questions and answers in a given chapter before proceeding to the next chapter.

6. Check the list of symbols or the glossary for any unfamiliar terms (Appendices C and D).

7. Take the Post-test after completing all the chapters (Appendix A).

8. Write me with any corrections, disagreements, suggestions for improvements, etc. If you have a personal computer, and want additional instruction in blood gas interpretation and respiratory failure management, consider the computer programs offered on the last page of this book.

Lawrence Martin, M.D.
Chief, Division of Pulmonary and
Critical Care Medicine
Mt. Sinai Medical Center
One Mt. Sinai Drive
Cleveland, Ohio 44106

Pre-test

Take this Pre-test now. If you answer over 90% of the 35 items correctly, give this book to a friend. You probably don't need it.

Directions: For each of the following seven statements or questions, there may be none, one, or more than one correct response. Circle the correct response(s) *before* checking the answers in Appendix B.

1. Normal range for $PaCO_2$ is 35-45 mm Hg. A change in $PaCO_2$ from normal to 28 mm Hg means the subject
   a) is hyperventilating.
   b) has excess alveolar ventilation for the amount of CO_2 production.
   c) must have hypoxia, anxiety, and/or metabolic acidosis.
   d) must be breathing faster than normal.
   e) must have acute respiratory alkalosis.

2. The arterial PO_2 is predicted to be reduced to some extent from
   a) anemia.
   b) ventilation-perfusion (V-Q) imbalance with an increase in the number of low V-Q units.
   c) increased PCO_2, while the subject is breathing room air.
   d) carbon monoxide poisoning.
   e) altitude.

3. To obtain a reasonable idea of the acid-base state of a patient's blood, you would need to know the
   a) pH and $PaCO_2$.
   b) pH and PaO_2.
   c) $PaCO_2$ and PaO_2.
   d) $PaCO_2$ and HCO_3^-.
   e) pH and SaO_2 (%saturation of hemoglobin with oxygen).

(continued)

4. Which of the following statements regarding acid-base balance (is) are correct?
   a) HCO_3^- increases with acute elevation of $PaCO_2$, before any renal compensation takes place.
   b) A patient can have metabolic acidosis and metabolic alkalosis at the same time.
   c) "Base excess" is normally zero +/- 2 mEq/L.
   d) An elevated "anion gap" is presumptive evidence for metabolic acidosis unless proven otherwise.
   e) In theory, the bicarbonate value calculated from the Henderson-Hasselbalch equation and the "CO_2" value measured in the chemistry lab as part of routine electrolyte measurements should be identical.

5. The following information is accurate and/or useful when determining a patient's arterial oxygen content (CaO_2).
   a) Each 100 ml of hemoglobin can combine with 1.34 ml of oxygen.
   b) Normal CaO_2 is between 16 and 22 mgm/dl.
   c) Normally, dissolved oxygen constitutes less than 2.0% of the CaO_2.
   d) Normally, mixed venous oxygen content at rest is about 25% less than CaO_2.
   e) A 10% decrease in SaO_2 will produce the same percentage decrease in CaO_2 as will a 10% decrease in hemoglobin content.

(continued)

PRE-TEST (CONTINUED)

6. Arterial blood gas data (pH, $PaCO_2$, PaO_2, SaO_2) are related in some simple but important ways. Which of the following are valid relationships?
   a) Alveolar PO_2 is related to $PaCO_2$ by the alveolar gas equation: as $PaCO_2$ goes up, alveolar PO_2 goes down.
   b) PaO_2 is inversely related to blood pH: as pH goes up, PaO_2 goes down.
   c) If $PaCO_2$ increases while HCO_3^- remains unchanged, pH always goes down.
   d) PaO_2 is related to SaO_2 on a linear scale (i.e., a straight-line relationship).
   e) The SaO_2 is related to hemoglobin-bound arterial oxygen content on a linear scale (i.e., a straight-line relationship).

7. There are some 'truisms' in terminology and physiology for proper blood gas interpretation. They include which of the following?
   a) "Hyperventilation" and "hypoventilation" are clinical terms, and are not diagnosed by arterial blood gases.
   b) The alveolar-arterial PO_2 difference increases with age and with increase in the fraction of inspired oxygen.
   c) The arterial PO_2 cannot go above 100 mm Hg while breathing room air at sea level.
   d) A continuously negative alveolar-arterial PO_2 difference is incompatible with life.
   e) If arterial pH is normal, the patient cannot have a clinically significant acid-base disorder.

END OF PRE-TEST

Introduction to Quik-Course on Blood Gas Interpretation

This book contains what anyone taking care of patients "really needs to know" about blood gas interpretation. The text, beginning on page 1, also includes many problems to help ensure your understanding of the material.

It is possible this amount of information may be more than you "really" want to study, at least for now. To accommodate those who want to begin with a quick review, or just don't have time to read the whole book right now, I have developed Quik-Course, an abbreviated syllabus on blood gas interpretation (Chapter 10).

Quik-Course includes the four major equations without in-depth explanations, omits all the problems and figures, and uses smaller type than the rest of the book. It is not "all" anyone needs to know but is a synopsis of the entire work. You can use Quik-Course as a starting point, as a final review, or as a refresher at any time.

The learning is up to you. Good luck!

CHAPTER 1.

What is Meant by Interpreting Arterial Blood Gases? One Blood Sample, Two Machines

One blood sample

This book is about how to interpret and use lab values obtained from a single arterial blood sample. Usually obtained from a radial, brachial or femoral artery, the blood is brought to the lab in a heparinized, ice-encased syringe, where it is promptly tested. Turnaround time from arterial blood drawing to results reporting is typically 10 to 20 minutes.

Strictly speaking, "blood gas" refers to any element or compound that is a gas under ordinary conditions and that is also dissolved to some extent in our blood. With this definition in mind, circle any of the following values that represent "blood gases." The terms are listed in alphabetical order. (Please make sure you circle your answers before reading further.)

?
a) base excess
b) bicarbonate
c) carbon dioxide
d) carbon monoxide
e) glucose
f) helium
g) hemoglobin
h) krypton
i) nitrogen
j) oxygen
k) pH

Carbon dioxide, carbon monoxide, helium, krypton, nitrogen and oxygen are gases under ordinary conditions and are also dissolved in our blood, hence they are all "blood gases." Although pH is not a gas, it is routinely measured with arterial blood gases and is now firmly fixed as part the "ABG test." Similarly, bicarbonate, not a blood gas but the anion of carbonic acid, is routinely calculated as part of every blood gas test. Base excess is a calculation that reflects how much acid or base is needed to normalize the total buffer base in the blood (see Chapter 6).

Although glucose is also dissolved in blood, it is not a gas but a granular material at room temperature. Similarly hemoglobin, the molecular carrier of oxygen within the red blood cell, is not a gas under any condition.

Nitrogen, krypton and helium are inert gases and are dissolved in our blood (the last two in trace amounts). Since inert gases cause no clinical problems, they are not measured as part of the arterial blood gas test. (Nitrogen can cause the bends and other difficulties in underwater diving, but such problems are a specialized area of medicine and in any case are not diagnosed with blood gas measurements.)

Carbon monoxide *is* a gas and is measured in its combined form with hemoglobin as percent carboxyhemoglobin (%COHb). Carbon monoxide *could* be measured in its dissolved state (as partial pressure of CO) but this component is minute and its measurement would only be an indirect guide to the %COHb, so %COHb is what the blood gas lab is set up to measure.

In summary, not all "blood gases" are routinely measured and not all "blood gas" measurements are of true blood gases. Carbon dioxide and oxygen are routinely measured as their partial pressures, $PaCO_2$ and PaO_2, respectively. Carbon monoxide, another blood gas, is measured as %COHb. Nitrogen, helium and krypton (as well as other inert blood gases) are not measured at all.

Two machines

In the lab, the syringe containing the arterial blood sample is taken out of the ice, its cap removed, and an aliquot of blood drawn up into the blood gas machine's sample chamber. *All* blood gas machines measure pH, $PaCO_2$ and PaO_2, and calculate (or allow for calculation of) the bicarbonate and base excess (Figure 1-1).*

Many hospital blood gas labs are also set up to run an aliquot of the arterial sample though *another* machine, called a co-oximeter (Figure 1-1). This machine measures SaO_2, %COHb, %methemoglobin, and hemoglobin content (in grams/dl). From this information the arterial oxygen content (CaO_2) can be calculated.

What is the maximum value attainable by adding the values obtained for SaO_2 + %COHb + %methemoglobin from a single blood sample?

?

a) 100%

b) 200%

b) depends on the hemoglobin content

Just as %COHb is the percent of hemoglobin sites chemically combined with carbon monoxide, SaO_2 is the percentage of hemoglobin sites chemically combined ("saturated") with oxygen, i.e., the $\%O_2Hb$ or %oxyhemoglobin (SaO_2 seems to be the more popular term). A hemoglobin-binding site cannot contain more

---

* This method is *in vitro*, since the blood samples are tested outside the body. In neonates and young children, PaO_2 is sometimes measured *in vivo* via a transcutaneous skin electrode, a technique rarely used in adults. Technology is also now available that allows continuous *in vivo* measurement of all three blood gas values — PaO_2, pH and $PaCO_2$ — through sensors inserted into the artery through an arterial catheter. Such improvements in technology may supplant *in vitro* analyses in critically ill patients, at least those who have indwelling arterial lines. The physiologic knowledge needed to interpret blood gas data, of course, should be the same regardless of the measuring technology.

than one gas molecule at the same time, so the two percentages (%O_2Hb and %COHb) are additive.

Methemoglobin is hemoglobin that has iron in its ferric or oxidized state (Fe^{+++}) as opposed to the normal ferrous state (Fe^{++}); hemoglobin with Fe^{+++} can bind *neither* oxygen nor carbon monoxide. Thus SaO_2, %COHb and %methemoglobin each represent separate portions of the total hemoglobin content and together cannot exceed 100%.

Figure 1-1. Two Blood Gas Machines: Measurements and Calculations (*).

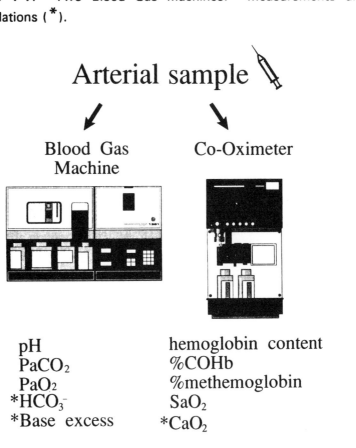

Arterial sample

Blood Gas Machine

Co-Oximeter

pH	hemoglobin content
$PaCO_2$	%COHb
PaO_2	%methemoglobin
*HCO_3^-	SaO_2
*Base excess	*CaO_2

In summary, the blood gas machine is used to measure partial pressure of oxygen and carbon dioxide (PO_2 and PCO_2) and pH and to perform some calculations based on this data. The co-oximeter is used to measure the various states and quantity of hemoglobin, values that allow for calculation of oxygen content (see Chapter 2). All blood gas labs are set up to measure PO_2, PCO_2 and pH; many labs also run the arterial sample through a co-oximeter to measure additional values (Figure 1-1). Normal values for blood gas measurements and calculations are shown in Table 1-1.

Table 1-1. Normal arterial blood gas values*

pH	7.35-7.45
$PaCO_2$	35-45 mm Hg
PaO_2	> 70 mm Hg**
HCO_3^-	22-26 mEq/L
%MetHb	<1%
%COHb	<2.5%
Base excess	-2.0 to 2.0 mEq/L
CaO_2	16-22 ml O_2/dl

* At sea level breathing ambient air

** Age-dependent

How much physiology do you need to know for proper blood gas interpretation?

No doubt about it, a knowledge of some basic pulmonary physiology is crucial to understanding arterial blood gas data. The next chapter will introduce the three physiologic processes and four equations important in blood gas interpretation.

Physiology textbooks teach the basics, but most of them don't relate the material to specific blood gas data or the clinical setting. However, without the basics you cannot build any clinical understanding. If you have a standard physiology textbook, you might want to review the sections on oxygenation, ventilation and acid-base as you work through this book. Texts particularly recommended for such review (if needed) are listed in the Bibliography (Appendix E). *All You Really Need To Know To Interpret Arterial Blood Gases* is predicated on basic physiology as taught in all medical schools (as well as in all respiratory therapy and four-year nursing schools). You are the best judge of whether additional review is necessary.

What other information is needed to interpret blood gas data?

In large part this book is about how to integrate blood gas values *with additional information*, in order to intelligently assess alveolar ventilation, oxygenation, and acid-base balance. When you can do that you will have learned to properly "interpret" blood gas data. In addition to some knowledge of basic pulmonary physiology, three areas of information are necessary for blood gas interpretation.

1. Information about the patient's immediate environment:
    fraction of inspired oxygen (FIO_2)
    barometric pressure

2. Additional lab data, for example:
    previous blood gas measurements
    electrolytes, blood sugar, BUN
    hemoglobin content or hematocrit
    chest x-ray
    pulmonary function tests

3. Clinical information. This includes the entire history and
    physical exam, with emphasis on the patient's:
    respiratory rate and other vital signs
    degree of respiratory effort
    mental status
    state of tissue perfusion

When confronted with blood gas data, always ask yourself: Do
I have the necessary clinical and laboratory information to
properly interpret these data? An isolated $PaCO_2$ reveals little
useful information without reference to the patient's mental status
and respiratory effort. A low PaO_2 may mean one thing if the
patient is inhaling supplemental oxygen, and quite another if the
patient is breathing room air. Similarly, knowledge of the chest
x-ray may be crucial to interpreting a low PaO_2. The pH and
HCO_3^- sometimes make sense only in light of the serum
electrolytes. To properly interpret blood gas data, you must know
the full clinical and laboratory picture.

The patient's environment: FIO_2 and barometric pressure

Normal PaO_2 is dependent on FIO_2 and barometric pressure,
as well as the patient's age. Air consists of a mixture of gases
containing approximately 21% oxygen, 78% nitrogen and 1% inert
gases, a composition that is unchanged throughout the breathable
atmosphere. At any altitude the fraction of inspired oxygen
(FIO_2) is 0.21. (FIO_2 is sometimes written as a percentage, e.g.,
21%. Either format is acceptable.)

Barometric pressure is a function of the weight of the atmosphere above the point of measurement. At sea level the barometric pressure averages 760 mm Hg, i.e., air pressure at sea level will sustain a closed column of mercury 760 mm high. The higher the altitude, the less weight of air at that point and the lower the barometric pressure. At the highest point on earth, the summit of Mt. Everest, barometric pressure is only 253 mm Hg (Figure 1-2).

Figure 1-2. Effects of altitude on barometric pressure (P_B). The height of the column of mercury supported by air decreases with increasing altitude due to the fall in P_B. In this figure PO_2 is the partial pressure of oxygen in dry air. Since $PO_2 = 0.21 \times P_B$, PO_2 also decreases with altitude. (From Martin L.: Pulmonary Physiology in Clinical Practice, Copyright 1987 by the C.V. Mosby Co., St. Louis.)

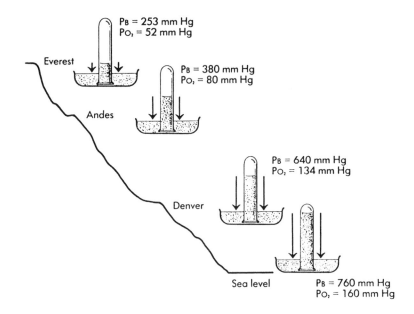

Barometric pressure is the sum of the pressures of all the constituent gases. Each gas exerts its own "partial pressure," which is the same pressure it would exert if no other gases were present. Table 1-2 shows the partial pressures for gases in dry air at sea level.

Table 1-2. Composition of dry air at sea level

	Percentage of gas in air	Sea level partial pressure (mm Hg)
Nitrogen	78.08	593.41
Oxygen	20.95	159.22
Carbon dioxide	00.03	.23
Other gases*	00.94	7.14
Total	100	760

*Mainly argon

The partial pressure of any gas in dry air is the percentage of gas in the air times the barometric pressure:

$$P_{GAS} \text{ in dry air} = \text{percentage of gas} \times P_B$$

Why *dry* air? Air often contains water vapor, which exerts its own partial pressure. To obtain the partial pressure of any gas such as oxygen or nitrogen, water vapor pressure must first be subtracted from the barometric pressure since it dilutes out all the dry gases. Depending on the climate, the amount of water vapor in ambient air varies from zero to fully saturated, and the partial pressure of water vapor from zero to over 50 mm Hg. For example, if ambient air is partly saturated so that P_{H20} is 27 mm Hg, then

$$P_{GAS} = \text{percentage of gas x } (P_B - 27 \text{ mm Hg}).$$

Regardless of the P_{H20} in ambient air, once air is inhaled it becomes fully saturated in the upper airway; hence all *inspired* air has a water vapor pressure of 47 mm Hg (at 98.6°F/37°C; water vapor pressure varies slightly with body temperature). For this reason, knowledge of the ambient air P_{H20} is not clinically important.

Table 1-2 lists the major gases in air and their partial pressures in dry air. Note that for clinical purposes we round off the percentage of oxygen in the air to .21 (21%); this is the FIO_2 or fraction of inspired oxygen when breathing ambient or "room" air. (Though there is a tiny amount of CO_2 in the atmosphere, for clinical purposes we assume an inspired PCO_2 of zero.)

Since the percentage of oxygen is constant throughout the breathable atmosphere, but the barometric pressure decreases with altitude, the pressure of oxygen must fall with altitude (Figure 1-2). To maintain acceptable oxygen levels at extreme altitude there are two broad options: change the environment or adapt physiologically.

The first option involves increasing either the FIO_2 or the barometric pressure. Airplane cabins are pressurized to around 6000 feet whenever planes fly higher than this altitude; this pressurization allows FIO_2 to be kept at .21 throughout the flight. Pressurization is of course not feasible out in the open. Mountain climbers carry portable oxygen to increase their FIO_2 at extreme altitudes (e.g., above 20,000 feet).

Physiologic adaptation, though well characterized for various altitudes, should not be relied upon at extremes of altitude. Nonetheless, as will be discussed in Chapter 4, it is physiologic adaptation that has allowed man to reach the summit of Mt. Everest *without supplemental oxygen.*

1-1. Two men first climbed the summit of Mt. Everest without supplemental oxygen in 1978. What major physiologic adaptation do you suppose makes such a climb possible?

One final point needs to be emphasized in discussing environmental pressures. The average *airway* pressure in the lungs will always equal the ambient or barometric pressure. (This is true during spontaneous breathing, i.e., without mechanical assistance.) When supplemental oxygen is breathed the extra oxygen displaces nitrogen from the body's tissues. The amount of nitrogen displaced depends on the FIO_2, but at any FIO_2 the total gaseous pressure remains atmospheric (i.e., equal to barometric pressure); oxygen pressure merely replaces the nitrogen pressure. Breathing 100% oxygen over a sufficient period of time will totally de-nitrogenate the tissues, a fact that becomes important in considering alveolar PO_2 (Chapter 4).

1-2. What is the average airway pressure of a:
a) Denver resident?
b) New Orleans resident?
c) climber in the Andes?
d) climber on the summit of Mt. Everest?
e) subject breathing air in a hyperbaric chamber pressurized to two atmospheres?

1-3. Denver is at one mile elevation (5280 feet). Assuming barometric pressure changes linearly with altitude, what is the dry air PO_2 in Leadville, Colorado (altitude 10200 feet), the highest incorporated city in the United States?

1-4. What is the total pressure of all gases in the lungs, apart from water vapor, under the following conditions:

a) P_B = 760 mm Hg, normal body temperature (37°C)?
b) P_B = 253 mm Hg, normal body temperature?
c) P_B = 760 mm Hg, body temperature 39°C? (Is it more or less than your answer for 1-4a?)

1-5. In general terms, what are the physiologic consequences during an airplane trip for someone traveling from the east coast to California, who:

a) is healthy, with PaO_2 95 mm Hg?
b) has mild chronic obstructive pulmonary disease (COPD), PaO_2 75 mm Hg?
c) has severe COPD, PaO_2 58 mm Hg?

Answers to numbered questions

1-1. The alveolar gas equation, introduced in the next chapter, shows that alveolar PO_2 is directly related to the inspired oxygen pressure and inversely related to the $PaCO_2$. The inspired oxygen pressure is fixed by the FIO_2 and barometric pressure. Mountain climbers adapt at altitude principally by lowering $PaCO_2$, thereby raising their alveolar (and arterial) PO_2.

1-2. The average airway pressure in any location equals the barometric pressure at that location (see Figure 1-2). Although the barometric pressure fluctuates slightly during the day, knowledge of the average barometric pressure at a particular altitude is sufficient for blood gas interpretation purposes. In Denver, average airway pressure is 640 mm Hg; in New Orleans, which is at sea level, 760 mm Hg. For the Andes the answer of course depends on the specific altitude in this mountain range, but 380 mm Hg is the barometric pressure (and hence the airway pressure) at some of the peaks. On the summit of Mt. Everest the barometric pressure has been measured at 253 mm Hg. Finally, in a hyperbaric chamber the ambient pressure is determined by the chamber; at two atmospheres the ambient pressure is

$$2 \times 760 \text{ mm Hg} = 1520 \text{ mm Hg},$$

which is also the average airway pressure of anyone in the chamber.

1-3. You are not expected to know the barometric pressure in Leadville, Colorado. However from Figure 1-2 you can figure out that P_B falls about 120 mm Hg per mile of altitude. Since Leadville is almost 2 miles high, that would give a P_B of about 520 mm Hg. Since FIO_2 is .21, the dry air PO_2 in Leadville is approximately 109 mm Hg (compared with 160 mm Hg at sea level).

Answers to numbered questions (continued)

1-4. a) Airway pressure = barometric pressure = 760 mm Hg. Water vapor pressure at 37°C = 47 mm Hg, which is subtracted to give the total gas pressure of 713 mm Hg (the sum of the partial pressures of oxygen, nitrogen and carbon dioxide in the lungs at sea level).

b) By the same reasoning as in 1-4(a), the total dry gas pressure is (253 - 47) mm Hg, or 206 mm Hg.

c) A febrile patient has a higher than normal water vapor pressure. At 39°C water vapor pressure is about 52.4 mm Hg, 5.4 mm Hg higher than normal; subtracting this value from barometric pressure of 760 mm Hg gives a dry gas pressure of about 707.6 mm Hg. (You are not expected to know the water vapor pressure at 39°C; a satisfactory answer to this question would have been "slightly lower than 713"). With most changes in body temperature, the change in dry gas pressure (sum of oxygen, nitrogen and carbon dioxide pressures) is trivial; for this reason water vapor pressure, for clinical purposes, is usually assumed to equal 47 mm Hg.

1-5. In all three examples the arterial PaO_2 can be expected to fall because of the drop in P_B, although the fall will be lessened by mild hyperventilation. Regardless of how high the plane flies, the fall in P_B is limited to a cabin pressure equal to about 6000 feet altitude, so the physiologic consequences for the healthy person are obviously insignificant. The drop in PaO_2 will be more significant for the patient with mild COPD, but it should pose no clinical problem if resting PaO_2 at sea level is 75 mm Hg. Patients with severe lung impairment, on the other hand, must be cautioned about airplane travel; a patient with PaO_2 in the 50s should either not fly or else receive supplemental oxygen en route, which can be provided by the airlines.

CHAPTER 2.

Three Physiologic Processes, Four Equations

Three physiologic processes

A student's first clinical exposure to arterial blood gases may be in the context of "let's check her PO_2," or "what's his PCO_2?" Certainly, a basic reason for the blood gas test is find out a patient's PaO_2, $PaCO_2$ or pH. But why do we want these values? What do they really tell us? In conjunction with other laboratory and clinical information, pH, PaO_2 and $PaCO_2$ help assess three vital physiologic processes:

- alveolar ventilation
- oxygenation
- acid-base balance

The only reason to obtain any blood gas measurement is to assess alveolar ventilation, oxygenation and/or acid-base balance. That is really what interpreting blood gases is all about. If there was a quicker and easier way to obtain this assessment, the arterial blood gas test would become obsolete.

Even if non-invasive methods become widely available for measuring pH, $PaCO_2$ and PaO_2 (as they have for SaO_2; see Chapter 5), there will still be a need for clinical interpretation. Methodology for laboratory tests changes frequently; the physiology of alveolar ventilation, oxygenation and acid-base balance is determined by nature and does not vary. For clinical purposes, the particular lab method that produces the data is not as important as understanding and using the information to benefit the patient.

Four Important Equations

Four basic equations are important for understanding and interpreting arterial blood gases:

	Physiologic process assessed
1. $PaCO_2$ equation	Alveolar ventilation
2. Alveolar gas equation	Oxygenation
3. Oxygen content equation	Oxygenation
4. Henderson-Hasselbalch equation	Acid-base balance

These equations are clinically useful not so much for the numbers they generate as for their *qualitative relationships*. It is not important that you memorize these equations now or ever. It *is* important that you learn the relationships among the variables they contain. As you read through the book and work on the problems, each equation and its clinical utility will become second nature to you. (Symbols used in these equations and elsewhere throughout the text are defined in Appendix C.)

1. *The PCO_2 equation* puts into physiologic perspective one of the most common of all clinical observations: a patient's respiratory rate and breathing effort. This equation states that alveolar PCO_2 ($PACO_2$) is directly proportional to the amount of CO_2 produced by metabolism and delivered to the lungs ($\dot{V}CO_2$), and inversely proportional to the alveolar ventilation ($\dot{V}A$). Because $PaCO_2$ can be assumed to equal $PACO_2$, this equation can be stated as follows:

$$PaCO_2 = \frac{\dot{V}CO_2 \times .863}{\dot{V}A}$$

where

PaCO$_2$ = arterial PCO$_2$ (mm Hg)

$\dot{V}$CO$_2$ = the amount of CO$_2$ produced by metabolism and delivered to the lungs (ml CO$_2$/min)

0.863 = constant that equates dissimilar units for $\dot{V}$CO$_2$ (ml CO$_2$/min) and $\dot{V}$A (L/min) to PaCO$_2$ pressure units (mm Hg)

$\dot{V}$A = alveolar ventilation (L/min) = $\dot{V}$E - $\dot{V}$D,
    where
    $\dot{V}$E = minute or total ventilation (L/min)
    $\dot{V}$D = dead space ventilation (L/min)

2-1. If CO$_2$ production stays the same and alveolar ventilation increases, PaCO$_2$ will

a) rise
b) fall
c) stay the same

2-2. If alveolar ventilation stays the same and CO$_2$ production increases, PaCO$_2$ will

a) rise
b) fall
c) stay the same

2-3. A patient running on a treadmill doubles her respiratory rate, pulse, rate of CO$_2$ production, minute and alveolar ventilation. If her baseline PaCO$_2$ is 40 mm Hg, her exercise PaCO$_2$ is

a) 20 mm Hg
b) 30 mm Hg
c) 40 mm Hg
d) impossible to determine

2-4.   A patient with severe emphysema has an FEV-1
second of 0.5 L (25% of predicted). His resting
$PaCO_2$ is 45 mm Hg. What will happen to his
$PaCO_2$ when he exercises if his minute and dead
space ventilation do not increase?

a) will increase along with increase in $\dot{V}CO_2$
b) will remain unchanged
c) will decrease due to exertional hyperventilation
d) change will depend on oxygen consumption

2. The *Alveolar gas equation* is essential to understanding any
PaO_2 value and in assessing if the lungs are properly transferring
oxygen into the blood. Is a PaO_2 of 28 mm Hg abnormal? How
about 50 mm Hg? 95 mm Hg? To understand *any* PaO_2 value
one also has to know the PCO_2, FIO_2 (fraction of inspired
oxygen) and the barometric pressure, all components of the
alveolar gas equation:

$$PAO_2 = PIO_2 - 1.2(PaCO_2)\ ^*$$

where
PAO_2 = mean alveolar PO_2 (mm Hg)
PIO_2 = partial pressure of inspired (tracheal) O_2 (mm Hg)
$\quad$ = FIO_2 (P_B - P_{H20})
$\quad\quad FIO_2$ = fraction of inspired oxygen (.XX)
$\quad\quad P_B$ = barometric pressure (mm Hg)
$\quad\quad P_{H20}$ = water vapor pressure (mm Hg)
$PaCO_2$ = arterial PCO_2 (mm Hg).

----

*   The equation presented here is widely used for clinical purposes. It is an
abbreviation of the formally derived alveolar gas equation:

$$PAO_2 = PIO_2 - (PACO_2) \left[FIO_2 + \frac{(1\text{-}FIO_2)}{R} \right]$$

As with the PCO_2 equation, PAO_2 is calculated assuming that $PaCO_2$ = $PACO_2$.

2-5. If PIO_2 stays the same and $PaCO_2$ increases, alveolar PO_2 will

   a) increase
   b) decrease
   c) remain the same

2-6. If $PaCO_2$ stays the same and FIO_2 increases, alveolar PO_2 will

   a) increase
   b) decrease
   c) remain the same

2-7. If sea level barometric pressure falls by half and the normal $PaCO_2$ falls by half, alveolar PO_2 will

   a) increase
   b) decrease
   c) remain the same

2-8. If PAO_2 increases above normal, PaO_2

   a) increases if the lungs are normal
   b) increases only if the lungs are normal and the patient is hyperventilating (has reduced $PaCO_2$)
   c) always increases

2-9. If PAO_2 decreases, PaO_2

   a) always decreases also
   b) decreases only if the lungs are abnormal
   c) decreases only if the lungs are abnormal and the patient is hypoventilating (has elevated $PaCO_2$)

Chapter 4 will discuss the relationship of PAO_2 to PaO_2 and clinical application of the "A-a O_2 difference."

3. Oxygen is a gas and exerts a pressure of course, but oxygen also has a content in the blood, notated CaO_2, with units ml O_2/dl blood. CaO_2 is calculated by the *oxygen content equation*:

$$CaO_2 = \text{amount of } O_2 \text{ bound to hemoglobin} + \text{amount of } O_2 \text{ dissolved in plasma}$$

$$CaO_2 = (SaO_2 \times Hb \times 1.34) + .003(PaO_2)$$

where

CaO_2 = ml O_2/dl arterial blood
SaO_2 = percent saturation of arterial hemoglobin with oxygen, expressed as decimal fraction (e.g., .98)
Hb = hemoglobin content (grams/dl blood)
1.34 = O_2-binding capacity of hemoglobin (ml O_2/gram hb)
.003 = solubility constant for dissolved O_2 in plasma
    = .003 ml O_2/dl/mm Hg PaO_2

Chapter 5 will explore in greater detail the difference between PaO_2 (oxygen pressure) and CaO_2 (oxygen content). Keep in mind that tissues require a certain amount of oxygen molecules delivered each minute, a need met by cardiac output and requisite oxygen content.

2-10.   If hemoglobin content decreases by 25%, CaO_2 will fall by

a) a lower percentage
b) a higher percentage
c) approximately the same percentage

2-11. If SaO_2 falls by 25%, CaO_2 will fall by

    a) approximately the same percentage
    b) a lower percentage
    c) a higher percentage

2-12. A doubling of PaO_2 from 50 mm Hg to 100 mm Hg, with no change in hemoglobin content, will

    a) double the CaO_2
    b) increase CaO_2 by more than 25%
    c) increase CaO_2 by less than 25%

2-13. If normal PaO_2 is 100 mm Hg and oxygen content is approximately 20 ml O_2/dl, approximately what percent of oxygen content is contributed by the dissolved fraction?

    a) 1.5%
    b) 3.0%
    c) 4.5%

2-14. If a patient's PaO_2 is 100 mm Hg but the oxygen content is only 10 ml O_2/dl (because of anemia), what percent is contributed by the dissolved fraction?

    a) 1.5%
    b) 3.0%
    c) 4.5%

4. The *Henderson-Hasselbalch equation* is perhaps the most familiar of the four used in basic blood gas interpretation. It relates pH to components of the bicarbonate buffer system, the largest such system in the extracellular fluid. Any blood acid-base disturbance is instantaneously reflected in one or both of its buffer components (HCO_3^- and $PaCO_2$); their ratio at any one

time determines the blood's acidity, as defined by pH in the H-H equation.

$$pH = pK + \log \frac{HCO_3^-}{0.03(PaCO_2)}$$

where
pH   = the negative logarithm of hydrogen ion concentration
pK   = 6.1, the negative logarithm of the dissociation constant
            for carbonic acid
HCO_3^- = the concentration of bicarbonate (mEq/L)
$PaCO_2$ = partial pressure of CO_2 in arterial blood (mm Hg)
0.03   = solubility coefficient for CO_2 in plasma
            (mEq/L/mm Hg)

   Because the H-H equation incorporates a logarithm, shortened versions have been promulgated for rapid calculation of $[H^+]$ and HCO_3^- (see Chapter 6). However, as with the other three equations, calculations are not as important as understanding the relationship among the variables.

   2-15.   If HCO_3^- and $PaCO_2$ double from their normal baseline value, pH will

         a) stay the same
         b) double
         c) depend on the change in pK of the buffer system

   2-16.   If HCO_3^- falls by half and $PaCO_2$ remains the same, pH will

         a) stay the same
         b) increase
         c) decrease

2-17. A pH of 7.40 means

a) HCO_3^- is normal
b) $PaCO_2$ is normal
c) the ratio of HCO_3^- to $PaCO_2$ is normal

2-18. If $PaCO_2$ increases from 40 to 60 mm Hg, the H-H equation predicts

a) pH will fall
b) bicarbonate will fall
c) bicarbonate will rise
d) nothing; change in a single variable cannot predict change in the other two

----

There are many other equations and formulas one can explore in a discussion of blood gas interpretation. The point is not to belabor equations but to emphasize *qualitative relationships* among key variables. Learn well the relationships expressed in these four equations and you will seldom, if ever, have to do any calculations.

With your pencil, complete the following statements.

2-19. If CO_2 production, PIO_2 and HCO_3^- remain constant, then as alveolar ventilation decreases _____ and _____ will also decrease.

2-20. If PIO_2 and HCO_3^- remain constant, then as $PaCO_2$ increases _____ and _____ will decrease.

2-21. The relationship of PaO$_2$ to CaO$_2$ has not been presented but you may already know it. How would you describe this relationship?

_____

_____

2-22. Changes in which of the following *will not* affect the PAO$_2$ (hint: stick to the equations):

a) PaCO$_2$
b) SaO$_2$
c) hemoglobin content
d) HCO$_3^-$
e) altitude
f) barometric pressure
g) FIO$_2$
h) patient's age

Write the four equations just presented in the spaces provided below, then check your responses by referring to the previous pages. Remember: *Correct expression of the relationships is more important than memorizing constants or doing the actual calculations.* Make sure you know the correct relationships for each equation before proceeding to Chapter 3.

PaCO$_2$ equation:

PaCO$_2$ =

Alveolar gas equation:

$PAO_2 =$

Oxygen content equation:

$CaO_2 =$

Henderson-Hasselbalch equation:

$pH =$

Answers to numbered questions

The questions in this chapter are designed to orient you to changes in relationships rather than mere quantitation. All can be answered with reference to one or more of the four equations presented.

2-1. Ans. b. The $PaCO_2$ equation states that $PaCO_2$ is directly related to CO_2 production and inversely related to alveolar ventilation. Hence if CO_2 production stays the same and alveolar ventilation increases, $PaCO_2$ has to fall.

2-2. Ans. a. With the same reasoning as in 2-1, if alveolar ventilation stays the same and CO_2 production increases, $PaCO_2$ will rise.

2-3. Ans. c. In this question the subject doubles her rate of CO_2 production *and* alveolar ventilation. Since both values double, her exercise $PaCO_2$ should remain unchanged at 40 mm Hg.

2-4. Ans. a. This question is qualitatively similar to No. 2-2. By definition a fixed minute and dead space ventilation means that alveolar ventilation is unchanged. Since CO_2 production increases with exercise, and alveolar ventilation (in this case) remains unchanged, $PaCO_2$ should increase. Note that oxygen consumption is not a variable in the $PaCO_2$ equation.

2-5. Ans. b. The alveolar gas equation states that PAO_2 goes up with increases in PIO_2 and down with increases in $PaCO_2$. Hence if PIO_2 remains the same and $PaCO_2$ increases, alveolar PO_2 will decrease.

2-6. Ans. a. If $PaCO_2$ stays the same and FIO_2 increases, alveolar PO_2 will increase.

Answers to numbered questions (continued)

2-7. Ans. b. In this example sea level barometric pressure (760 mm Hg) and baseline $PaCO_2$ (40 mm Hg) each fall by half. A fall in P_B will lower, whereas a fall in $PaCO_2$ will raise, the alveolar PO_2. A brief calculation shows that, percentage-wise, reducing $PaCO_2$ cannot compensate for decreases in barometric pressure. In this example PAO_2 will decrease.

2-8. Ans. a. When PAO_2 increases, PaO_2 will also increase if the lungs are normal. This occurs whether or not the person with normal lungs hyperventilates, hence answer b is incorrect. If the lungs are diseased, PaO_2 may not go up with increases in PAO_2, hence answer c is incorrect.

2-9. Ans. a. Since oxygen enters the blood only by passive diffusion, PAO_2 defines the upper limit of PaO_2. Any decrease of PAO_2 will be reflected in a decrease of PaO_2. Note that the opposite is not true, since the lower limit of PaO_2 is determined by the state of the lungs (ventilation-perfusion relationships).

2-10. Ans. c. If hemoglobin content decreases by 25%, CaO_2 will fall by approximately the same percentage ("approximately" because the dissolved O_2 fraction, which accounts for very little of the oxygen content, will not change as hemoglobin falls).

2-11. Ans. a. Reasoning as in 2-10.

2-12. Ans. c. Doubling PaO_2 from 50 mm Hg to 100 mm Hg, with no change in hemoglobin content, will change the CaO_2 according to the change in the variables in the O_2 content equation. PaO_2 values of 50 mm Hg and 100 mm Hg represent an oxygen saturation of about 85% and 98%, respectively. Hence CaO_2 will increase by less than 25%.

2-13. Ans. a. Since dissolved fraction = .003 ml O_2/dl x PaO_2, the amount of dissolved oxygen is .3 ml/dl. This comes to 1.5% of the total.

Answers to numbered questions (continued)

2-14. Ans. b. Since the PaO_2 is the same as in problem 2-13, the dissolved component .3 ml O_2/dl. However, since the oxygen content is only 10 ml O_2/dl, half that in problem 2-13, the percentage contributed by dissolved oxygen is double, or 3%.

2-15. Ans. a. The H-H equation states that pH is directly related to the ratio of HCO_3^- over $PaCO_2$. Hence if HCO_3^- and $PaCO_2$ double from their normal baseline value their ratio, and the resulting pH, will stay the same.

2-16. Ans. c. If HCO_3^- falls by half and $PaCO_2$ remains the same, pH will decrease.

2-17. Ans. c. A pH of 7.40 means only that the *ratio* of HCO_3^- to $PaCO_2$ is normal.

2-18. Ans. d. The H-H equation, per se, predicts nothing from a change in only one variable. Although acute CO_2 retention is manifested by a reduced pH and slight elevation of HCO_3^-, these changes are not predicted by the equation.

2-19. Based on the equations presented in this chapter, if CO_2 production, PIO_2, and HCO_3^- remain constant, then as alveolar ventilation decreases, *pH* and *PAO_2* will also decrease.

2-20. If PIO_2 and HCO_3^- remain constant, then as $PaCO_2$ increases, *pH* and *PAO_2* will decrease.

2-21. The relation of PaO_2 to CaO_2 is the same as the relation of PaO_2 to SaO_2, i.e., a sigmoid-shaped curve.

2-22. Changes in the following parameters will *not* affect the PAO_2: SaO_2; hemoglobin content; HCO_3^-; patient's age. $PaCO_2$, barometric pressure, altitude (through its effect on barometric pressure) and FIO_2 are variables in the alveolar gas equation and so will affect the PAO_2.

CHAPTER 3.

$PaCO_2$ and Alveolar Ventilation

High and low $PaCO_2$

As with any single laboratory value, $PaCO_2$ can be either high or low. Since normal $PaCO_2$ is 35-45 mm Hg, a $PaCO_2$ > 45 mm Hg is "high" and < 35 mm Hg is "low." Of course proper interpretation of $PaCO_2$ is somewhat more sophisticated (or you wouldn't be reading this book!).

In discussing $PaCO_2$ there should be some agreement on terminology. "Hypercapnia" and "hypocapnia" are the terms for high and low $PaCO_2$, respectively. The *opposite* prefix denotes the respective state of alveolar ventilation.

$PaCO_2$	Condition in blood	State of alveolar ventilation
> 45 mm Hg	Hypercapnia	Hypoventilation
35 - 45 mm Hg	Eucapnia	Normal ventilation
< 35 mm Hg	Hypocapnia	Hyperventilation

The reason *hyper*capnia reflects a state of *hypo*ventilation is shown by the $PaCO_2$ equation, first introduced in Chapter 2:

$$PaCO_2 = \frac{\dot{V}CO_2 \text{ x } .863}{\dot{V}A}$$

Alveolar ventilation ($\dot{V}A$) is the total amount of air breathed per minute ($\dot{V}E$; expired or minute ventilation) *minus* that air which goes to dead space per minute ($\dot{V}D$).

$$\dot{V}A = \dot{V}E - \dot{V}D$$

where

$\dot{V}E$ = respiratory rate x tidal volume

$\dot{V}D$ = respiratory rate x dead space volume

Figure 3-1 is a schematic of the lungs showing separation of dead space and alveolar space, and their respective ventilations. Figures like this one, often reproduced in textbooks, suggest the volumes are fixed, although they are not. The dead space volume (150 ml in the figure) represents non-ventilating airways (the upper airway, bronchi and bronchioles), but alveoli can be *converted into* dead space when they are unperfused, as commonly happens in many lung diseases.

Thus there are really two dead space volumes: anatomic and physiologic. Anatomic dead space includes all the airways that anatomically can never take part in gas exchange, i.e., all airways down to the alveolar level. Physiologic dead space includes all the anatomic dead space *plus* alveolar spaces that receive air but do not participate in gas exchange (generally because they are underperfused).

Since all alveoli normally take part in gas exchange the distinction between the two dead spaces is not so important in the healthy individual. In various pulmonary diseases, physiologic dead space can greatly exceed anatomic dead space. The normal ratio of physiologic dead space to tidal volume is about one-third, or 167 ml for a tidal volume of 500 ml.

The dead space in the $PaCO_2$ equation is the physiologic dead space. The symbol, $\dot{V}D$, thus represents the amount of air entering the physiologic dead space per minute, i.e., *all* the air that does not take part in gas exchange. Note that air which enters alveoli but doesn't exchange gases is just as "wasted" as the air entering the trachea and bronchi.

Figure 3-1. Schematic of the lungs showing the difference between lung volumes and ventilations. See text for further discussion. (From Martin L.: Pulmonary Physiology in Clinical Practice, Copyright 1987 by the C.V. Mosby Co., St. Louis.)

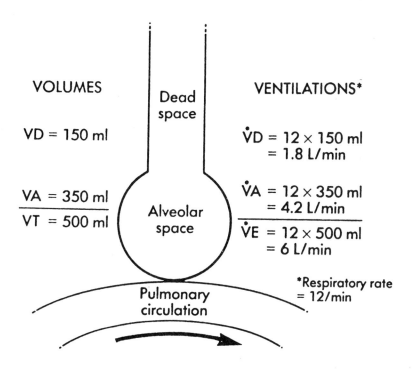

In lung diseases characterized by altered ventilation-perfusion ratios, physiologic dead space can be large. In emphysema, for example, physiologic dead space can exceed 50% or even 60% of the patient's tidal volume. Such patients have to work very hard to bring air to gas-exchanging alveoli.

> 3-1.   What are the dead space volume and $\dot{V}D$ if tidal volume is 500 ml, respiratory rate = 12/minute, and $\dot{V}A$ = 3 L/min?
>
> 3-2.   Does this volume represent anatomic or physiologic dead space?

From the $PaCO_2$ equation it is evident that hypoventilation resulting in elevated $PaCO_2$ is really "hypo*alveolar*ventilation relative to CO_2 production." Similarly, hyperventilation leading to low $PaCO_2$ is really "hyper*alveolar*ventilation relative to CO_2 production." By convention, the terms "alveolar" and "relative to CO_2 production" are omitted when characterizing the state of ventilation as it relates to $PaCO_2$.

Notice that the *only* number needed for determining the patient's state of alveolar ventilation is the $PaCO_2$. We do not need to know the actual amount of alveolar ventilation or CO_2 production (they are not routine measurements and are never reported with routine blood gas values).

Clinically, we need to know only *if* a patient's $\dot{V}A$ is adequate for $\dot{V}CO_2$; if it is, then $PaCO_2$ will be in the normal range (35-45 mm Hg). Conversely, a normal $PaCO_2$ means only that alveolar ventilation is adequate for the patient's level of CO_2 production at the moment $PaCO_2$ was measured.

In summary, the terms hypo- and hyperventilation refer only to high or low $PaCO_2$, respectively. For reasons that will be discussed subsequently, these terms should not be used to characterize any patient's rate or depth of respirations, or the work of breathing.

3-3.   What is the PaCO$_2$ of a patient with respiratory rate 24/min, tidal volume 300 ml, dead space volume 150 ml, CO$_2$ production 300 ml/min? The patient shows some evidence of respiratory distress.

3-4.   Is the patient in the above problem hyper-, hypo-, or ventilating normally?

3-5.   What is the PaCO$_2$ of a patient with respiratory rate 10/min, tidal volume 600 ml, dead space volume 150 ml, CO$_2$ production 200 ml/min? The patient shows some evidence of respiratory distress.

3-6.   Is the patient described in problem 3-5 hyper-, hypo- or ventilating normally?

3-7.   Which of the following patients can be said to be hyperventilating?

   a) 50-year-old man with respiratory rate 30/min, using accessory muscles of breathing.

   b) A comatose 29-year-old woman with respiratory rate 8/min, PaCO$_2$ 28 mm Hg.

   c) A 65-year-old man with tidal volume 400 ml, respiratory rate 22/min.

*   *   *

Read the following statement and decide whether it is true or false before continuing:

?

The *only* physiologic reason for elevated PaCO$_2$ is a level of alveolar ventilation inadequate for the amount of CO$_2$ produced and delivered to the lungs. TRUE or FALSE?

Since $PaCO_2$ equals CO_2 production over alveolar ventilation — and nothing else — this is a true statement. Note the emphasis on inadequate alveolar ventilation as opposed to excess CO_2 production. This is because excess CO_2 production is not a problem for the normal respiratory system.

If excess CO_2 production were to cause hypercapnia, you would expect to see it during exercise, where the greatest rates of CO_2 production occur. During submaximal exercise (below the point of anaerobic metabolism), $PaCO_2$ stays in the normal range because $\dot{V}A$ rises proportional to the rise in $\dot{V}CO_2$. With extremes of exercise (beyond the anaerobic threshold), $PaCO_2$ *falls* as compensation for the developing lactic acidosis. In a healthy individual, $PaCO_2$ may be reduced (normal hyper-ventilation) but it is never elevated.

With the understanding that the physiologic basis for all hypercapnia is alveolar ventilation inadequate for CO_2 production, you can now appreciate the clinical reasons for an elevated $PaCO_2$. Since $\dot{V}A = \dot{V}E - \dot{V}D$, *any* elevated $PaCO_2$ can be explained by one of the following situations:

a) NOT ENOUGH $\dot{V}E$. This may occur from central nervous system depression (e.g., drug overdose), respiratory muscle paralysis (e.g., myasthenia gravis), or any other condition that affects rate or depth of breathing.

b) TOO MUCH OF THE $\dot{V}E$ ENDING UP AS $\dot{V}D$. This commonly occurs in severe chronic obstructive pulmonary disease where the architecture of alveolar spaces is altered, so that alveoli are ventilated but unperfused or under perfused. The result is an excess of physiologic dead space. Excess $\dot{V}D$ can also occur when the breathing is rapid and shallow, sometimes seen in severe restrictive impairment (e.g., pulmonary fibrosis).

c) SOME COMBINATION OF a) AND b). This may occur, for example, in a patient with both severe COPD and muscle fatigue. The COPD gives an increase in $\dot{V}D$ while the fatigue makes it difficult for the patient to sustain an adequate minute ventilation.

Assessing ventilation at the bedside

An important clinical corollary of the PaCO$_2$ equation is that one cannot reliably assess the adequacy of alveolar ventilation, and hence PaCO$_2$, at the bedside. $\dot{V}E$ can be easily measured with a handheld spirometer (as tidal volume times respiratory rate), but there is no way to know the amount of $\dot{V}E$ going to dead space *or* the patient's rate of CO$_2$ production. A common mistake is to assume that because someone is breathing fast, hard and/or deep they are "hyperventilating." Not so, of course.

> CASE. An intern is called to the bedside of an elderly woman patient late at night. She is anxious and complains of shortness of breath during examination. Lung fields are clear to auscultation and vital signs are normal except for slight tachycardia and respiratory rate 30/minute. A nurse comments that the patient "gets like this every night." The physician orders an anti-anxiety drug for what he describes as "hyperventilation and anxiety." Thirty minutes later the patient's breathing slows considerably and she becomes cyanotic, whereupon she is transferred to the intensive care unit.

What would you guess were this patient's blood gas values prior to receiving the anti-anxiety drug?

?
a) PaCO$_2$ 32 mm Hg, PaO$_2$ 60 mm Hg
b) PaCO$_2$ 43 mm Hg, PaO$_2$ 80 mm Hg
c) PaCO$_2$ 58 mm Hg, PaO$_2$ 52 mm Hg

Although nothing in the PCO_2 equation directly relates respiratory rate or depth of breathing to $PaCO_2$, such observations are commonly (and mistakenly) used to assess a patient's $PaCO_2$. The error in this case was to assume the patient was hyperventilating (because she was breathing fast) and could tolerate the sedative; in fact she was most likely hypoventilating and hypoxemic (answer c).

Hypercapnia represents a failure of some component of the respiratory system (comprised of the central nervous system, thoracic cage including the diaphragm, and lungs and airways), and therefore a state of advanced organ system impairment. Clinically, the problem could range from stable COPD to acute pulmonary edema; the patient could be in no distress or in need of emergency resuscitation.

In addition to the clinical implications of hypercapnia, there are three physiologic reasons why elevated $PaCO_2$ is potentially dangerous. First, as $PaCO_2$ increases, PAO_2 (and PaO_2) will fall unless inspired oxygen is supplemented (see Chapter 4). Second, as $PaCO_2$ increases, unless HCO_3^- also increases, pH will fall (see Chapter 6). Third, the higher the $PaCO_2$, the less defended is the patient against any further decline in $\dot{V}A$.

This last point is graphically illustrated by plotting $PaCO_2$ against alveolar ventilation (Figure 3-2). The higher the $PaCO_2$ to begin with, the more it will rise for any given decrement in $\dot{V}A$. For example, when $\dot{V}CO_2$ is 200 ml/min, a decrease in $\dot{V}A$ of 1 L/min (as may occur from anesthesia, sedation, pneumonia, and other causes) will increase a patient's baseline $PaCO_2$ of 29 mm Hg to 34.5 mm Hg. The same 1 L/min decline in alveolar ventilation will raise a baseline PCO_2 of 60 mm Hg to 90 mm Hg.

Figure 3-2. PaCO$_2$ vs. alveolar ventilation (V̇A). The relationship is shown for carbon dioxide production rates of 200 ml/min and 300 ml/min. A decrease in alveolar ventilation in the hypercapnic patient will result in a greater rise in PaCO$_2$ than the same V̇A change when PaCO$_2$ is low or normal. Also, an increase in carbon dioxide production when V̇A is fixed will result in an increase in PaCO$_2$. (From Martin L.: **Pulmonary Physiology in Clinical Practice,** Copyright 1987 by the C.V. Mosby Co., St. Louis.)

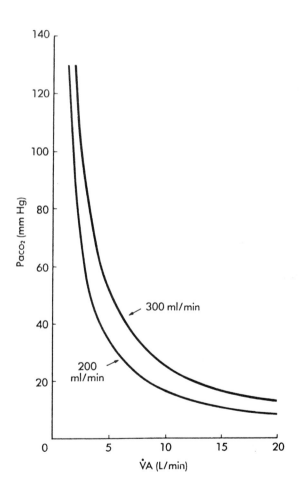

3.8 Given a $\dot{V}CO_2$ of 300 ml/min, what change in $PaCO_2$ will result from a 1 L/min decrease in $\dot{V}A$ when baseline $PaCO_2$ is

    a) 30 mm Hg
    b) 40 mm Hg
    c) 50 mm Hg

3.9 Given a fixed alveolar ventilation of 4 L/min, calculate the $PaCO_2$ for each of the following rates of CO_2 production.

    a) 200 ml/min
    b) 300 ml/min
    c) 400 ml/min

3.10 A severely emphysematous patient is exercised on a treadmill at 3 miles/hr. His rate of CO_2 production increases by 50% but he is unable to augment alveolar ventilation. If his resting $PaCO_2$ is 40 mm Hg and resting $\dot{V}CO_2$ is 200 ml/min, what will be his *exercise* $PaCO_2$?

Non-invasive measurement of PCO_2

Because carbon dioxide is never diffusion limited, alveolar PCO_2 ($PACO_2$) is assumed equal to $PaCO_2$. In theory, measurement of $PACO_2$ could substitute for $PaCO_2$, although in practice this is not always the case.

Figure 3-3 shows a normal tracing of expired PCO_2, measured during a tidal volume breath with an infrared CO_2 analyzer. The first part of the expired air is the same as the last part that was *inspired* on the previous breath (it is dead space air from the upper airways and will contain almost no carbon dioxide).

Figure 3-3. End-tidal carbon dioxide measurements. (From Martin
L.: Pulmonary Physiology in Clinical Practice, Copyright 1987 by the
C.V. Mosby Co., St. Louis.)

A. A single expired breath from a healthy subject, the end-tidal
point reflects alveolar, and hence arterial, partial pressure of CO_2.

B. Continuous monitoring of end-tidal carbon dioxide (PetCO₂) in a
patient with severe chronic obstructive pulmonary disease. Some
variation is seen during quiet breathing but average PetCO₂ is about
50 mm Hg. The PaCO₂ measured at the same time was 74 mm Hg.

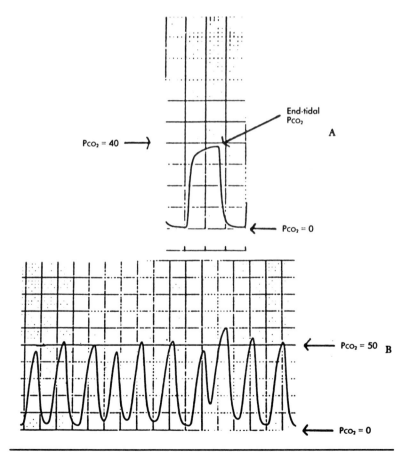

Gradually, air from some of the alveoli begins to join this dead space air, and the PCO_2 rises. By the very end of exhalation, all the dead space air has left the lungs, and the last few milliliters of air are from the alveoli only. This tracing shows that the end-tidal PCO_2 ($PetCO_2$) is approximately 38 mm Hg, which is the same as alveolar PCO_2 and therefore indicates a normal $PaCO_2$.

$PetCO_2$ can be measured on a continuous basis with modern capnographers, but the measurement has limitations. One has to assure that the carbon dioxide cannula, which delivers the expired air to the carbon dioxide analyzer, is not contaminated with room air. This is not so much of a problem with intubated patients (the cannula is inserted in the ventilator's expiratory circuit) as it is in other patients.

Perhaps the major pitfall is the difficulty of obtaining true $PACO_2$ in patients with severe lung disease. In many lung diseases, $PetCO_2$ may not reflect alveolar and arterial PCO_2, because of ventilation-perfusion imbalance and a resulting large increase in physiologic dead space. Because of the admixture of dead space air (PCO_2 almost zero) with alveolar air in the measured sample, the $PetCO_2$ in patients with increased dead space will always be *lower* than $PACO_2$.

In the example shown in Figure 3-3, from a patient with severe COPD, the $PetCO_2$ averaged approximately 50 mm Hg but $PaCO_2$ was 74 mm Hg, for a $PaCO_2$-$PetCO_2$ difference of 24 mm Hg. In this situation, the diseased alveoli do not empty evenly, and the end-tidal sample still reflects considerable dead space air.

A large $PaCO_2$-$PetCO_2$ difference does not obviate the value of the end-tidal measurement for physiologic monitoring; a rise in $PetCO_2$ still suggests a rise in $PaCO_2$, but one cannot equate the measured $PetCO_2$ with $PaCO_2$. For physiologic monitoring of critically ill patients, one or two comparisons should be made between $PetCO_2$ and $PaCO_2$ before following the $PetCO_2$ trend.

The absolute value of the $PaCO_2$-$PetCO_2$ difference has also been advocated for diagnostic purposes, especially in acute pulmonary embolism where the value is often much higher than in chronic lung conditions. The pulmonary embolus creates extra dead space by blocking perfusion to a group of alveoli. Air reaches these alveoli but does not take part in gas exchange because perfusion to them is blocked by the embolus. Although elegant in theory, this measurement is not generally used in clinical practice because of its lack of specificity.

$PaCO_2$ — Its relationship to oxygenation and acid-base balance

Any discussion of gas exchange and arterial blood gases should begin with $PaCO_2$. $PaCO_2$ is the only blood gas value that provides information on ventilation, oxygenation and acid-base balance. Figure 3-4 shows the relationship of $PaCO_2$ to:

- alveolar ventilation, in the $PaCO_2$ equation (as discussed in this chapter),

- PAO_2, in the alveolar gas equation (see Chapter 4), and

- pH, in the Henderson-Hasselbalch equation (see Chapter 6).

$PaCO_2$ is the "key" to understanding arterial blood gases in clinical practice. Understand $PaCO_2$ and all its ramifications — difference between alveolar and minute ventilation, determinants of hyper- and hypoventilation, how $PaCO_2$ figures in the alveolar gas and H-H equations — and you will be well on your way to mastering arterial blood gas interpretation.

Figure 3-4. $PaCO_2$ in ventilation, oxygenation, and acid-base equations. An elevated $PaCO_2$ indicates diminished $\dot{V}A$ relative to $\dot{V}CO_2$, and will result in a fall in PAO_2 (and hence PaO_2) and pH.

$$PaCO_2 = \frac{\dot{V}CO_2 \times .863}{\dot{V}A}$$

$$PAO_2 = PIO_2 - 1.2(PaCO_2) \qquad pH = 6.1 + \log \frac{HCO_3^-}{.03(PaCO_2)}$$

Answers to numbered questions

3-1. The $\dot{V}E$ or minute ventilation is 12 x 500 = 6 L/min. We are told that $\dot{V}A$ = 3 L/min. Hence $\dot{V}D = \dot{V}E - \dot{V}A$ = 3 L/min. The dead space volume is one-twelfth of the dead space ventilation, or 250 ml.

3-2. Alveolar ventilation is that part of total ventilation which reaches the alveoli *and* takes part in gas exchange. By definition, what's left includes all the air that enters the airways and does not take part in gas exchange, a volume that comprises the *physiologic* dead space.

3-3. First, you must calculate the alveolar ventilation. Since minute ventilation is 24 x 300 or 7.2 L/min, and dead space ventilation is 24 x 150 or 3.6 L/min, alveolar ventilation is 3.6 L/min. Then

$$PaCO_2 = \frac{\dot{V}CO_2 \times .863}{\dot{V}A}$$

$$PaCO_2 = \frac{300 \text{ ml/min} \times .863}{3.6 \text{ L/min}}$$

$$PaCO_2 = 71.9 \text{ mm Hg}$$

3-4. This patient is definitely hypoventilating.

Answers to numbered questions (continued)

3-5. $\dot{V}A = \dot{V}E - \dot{V}D$
        $= 10(600) - 10(150)$
        $= 6 - 1.5 = 4.5 \text{ L/min}$

$$PaCO_2 = \frac{200 \text{ ml/min} \times .863}{4.5 \text{ L/min}} = 38.4 \text{ mm Hg}$$

3-6.   This patient has normal alveolar ventilation for the rate of CO_2 production. However, the appearance of respiratory distress suggests the patient is trying to hyperventilate but can't, a potentially dangerous situation.

3-7.   Of the examples presented, you have only enough information to state that patient b) is hyperventilating. The other two patients *may* be hyperventilating but they might *also* be hypoventilating. Respiratory rate, tidal volume and use of accessory muscles are not sufficient information to make this determination.

3.8   You could obtain the requested information from the graph in Figure 3.2 or calculate $PaCO_2$ using the $PaCO_2$ equation in each situation. The answers below are from actual calculations.

        a) 30 mm Hg, $\dot{V}A = 8.63$ L/min. A decrease in $\dot{V}A$ to 7.63 L/min will give a $PaCO_2$ of 33.0 mm Hg (an increase of 3 mm Hg).

        b) 40 mm Hg, $\dot{V}A = 6.47$ L/min. A decrease of $\dot{V}A$ to 5.47 L/min will give a $PaCO_2$ of 47.3 mm Hg (an increase of 7.3 mm Hg).

Answers to numbered questions (continued)

3-8.　c) 50 mm Hg, $\dot{V}A = 5.18$ L/min. A decrease of $\dot{V}A$ to 4.18 L/min will give a $PaCO_2$ of 61.9 mm Hg (an increase of 11.9 mm Hg).

3-9.　In this question, alveolar ventilation is fixed at 4 liters/minute; $PaCO_2$ for different rates of CO_2 production are calculated using the $PaCO_2$ equation.

　　　a) 200 ml/min; $PaCO_2 = 43.2$ mm Hg
　　　b) 300 ml/min; $PaCO_2 = 64.7$ mm Hg
　　　c) 400 ml/min; $PaCO_2 = 86.3$ mm Hg

3-10.　Exercise increases CO_2 production. People with a normal respiratory system are always able to augment alveolar ventilation to meet or exceed the amount of $\dot{V}A$ necessary to excrete any excess CO_2 production. As in this example, patients with severe COPD or other forms of chronic lung disease are often *not* able to increase their alveolar ventilation. This patient's resting alveolar ventilation is

$$\frac{20 \text{ ml/min} \times .863}{40 \text{ mm Hg}} = 4.32 \text{ L/min}$$

Since he increased CO_2 production by 50% and alveolar ventilation not at all, his new $PaCO_2$ is

$$\frac{300 \text{ ml/min} \times .863}{4.32 \text{ L/min}} = 59.9 \text{ mm Hg}$$

CHAPTER 4.

PaO$_2$ and the Alveolar-arterial PO$_2$ Difference

Mean alveolar PO$_2$ and the alveolar gas equation

The principal function of the lungs is to exchange oxygen and carbon dioxide with the atmosphere. The lungs take in fresh air, a mixture of 21% oxygen, 78% nitrogen and trace carbon dioxide, and exhale stale air, a mixture of 17% oxygen, the same amount of nitrogen and about 4% carbon dioxide (Figure 4-1).

Only CO$_2$ and O$_2$ participate in gas exchange; there is no net exchange for nitrogen or other inert gases. Exchange of CO$_2$ and O$_2$ takes place through the alveolar-capillary membrane by passive diffusion, from a region of relatively higher gas pressure to one of relatively lower gas pressure (Figure 4-2). (In the early 1900s there was debate about whether gas exchange involved active transport; experiments at various altitudes showed passive diffusion is the only physiologic process involved).

Since O$_2$ enters the pulmonary capillary blood by diffusion, alveolar PO$_2$ must be a major determinant of pulmonary capillary and arterial PO$_2$. By the same reasoning, PAO$_2$ defines the upper limit of PaO$_2$; PaO$_2$ can never be higher than PAO$_2$. In the so-called "ideal" lung PaO$_2$ would equal PAO$_2$. However, gas exchange is not ideal and so PaO$_2$ should *always be less* than the calculated PAO$_2$. The actual difference between calculated PAO$_2$ and measured PaO$_2$ depends on several factors, the most important of which is the relationship of ventilation to perfusion among the hundreds of million alveolar-capillary units.

Figure 4-1. Gas exchange within the lungs. The lungs take in fresh air, a mixture of 21% O_2, 78% N_2 and trace CO_2. Exhaled air is a mixture of 17% O_2, the same percentage of N_2 inhaled, and 4% CO_2. The difference between inhaled and exhaled O_2 and CO_2 represents gas exchange with the atmosphere.

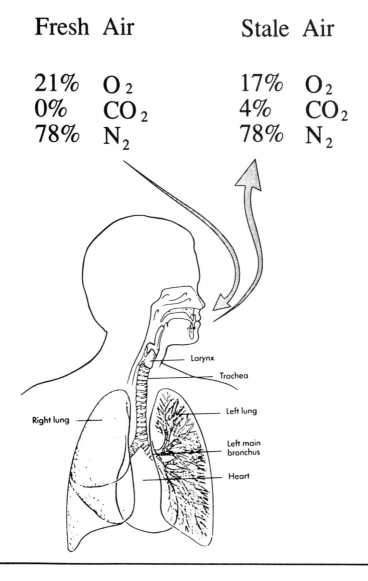

Figure 4-2. O_2 and CO_2 are exchanged through the alveolar-capillary membrane by diffusion from a region of relatively higher gas pressure to one of relatively lower gas pressure. In this figure, the difference between PCO_2 in blood entering the pulmonary capillary (mixed venous) and in the alveolus is 6 mm Hg. The difference between PO_2 in blood entering the pulmonary capillary and alveolus is 62 mm Hg. Note that end-capillary PO_2 and PCO_2 are identical to the alveolar PO_2 and PCO_2, respectively. (From Martin L.: Pulmonary Physiology in Clinical Practice, Copyright 1987 by the C.V. Mosby Co., St. Louis.)

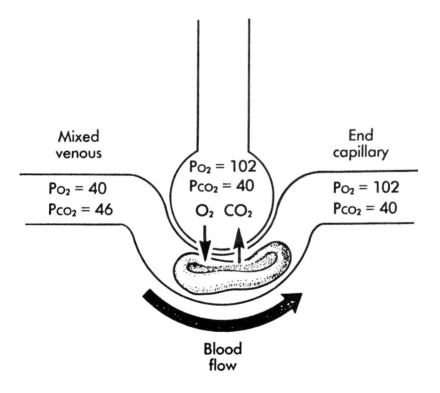

There are several hundred million individual alveoli. The PO_2 within their air spaces is not uniform, mainly because of effects of gravity and compliance (in upright humans, compliance or distensibility of the lungs is lowest at the apices and highest at the bases). For clinical purposes we don't have to concern ourselves with the distribution of individual alveolar PO_2 values. We only need to know the average PO_2 of *all* the alveoli, a value obtained by the alveolar gas equation:

$$PAO_2 = PIO_2 - 1.2(PaCO_2)$$

where

$$PIO_2 = FIO_2(P_B - 47).$$

The alveolar gas equation states that the average alveolar PO_2 equals the inspired PO_2 minus the arterial PCO_2 (times 1.2). Although the alveolar gas equation is formally derived using *alveolar* PCO_2, we assume that $PaCO_2 = PACO_2$ (as with the PCO_2 equation).

The factor 1.2 accounts for the slight variation in nitrogen pressure as more O_2 is taken up than CO_2 exhaled; the ratio of O_2 uptake to CO_2 exhaled is called the respiratory quotient and (for clinical purposes) is assumed to be 0.8. It is not necessary to measure RQ in the clinical setting. A recent study has confirmed the validity of this assumption for most patients (Cinel 1991).

With increasing FIO_2, the multiplication factor decreases because nitrogen is being eliminated from the body. With complete de-nitrogenation of the alveoli and blood (by breathing 100% oxygen), the multiplication factor becomes 1.0. In clinical practice you can use the factor 1.2 up to an FIO_2 of 0.6, and then 1.0 at 0.6 or higher (Martin 1986).

In the calculation of PIO_2, water vapor pressure (47 mm Hg) is subtracted from barometric pressure to give dry gas pressure. Water vapor pressure changes slightly with body temperature but the change is rarely enough to matter when calculating a patient's PAO_2.

Ambient FIO_2 is 0.21 (or 21%) at all altitudes. For patients breathing supplemental oxygen, the correct FIO_2 must be known to obtain an accurate PAO_2. However, it is usually not necessary to measure barometric pressure (P_B) if you know its approximate average value where the blood was drawn (e.g., sea level 760 mm Hg; Cleveland 747 mm Hg; Denver 640 mm Hg). This assumption facilitates calculation of PAO_2 because, for a given location, you can always use the same value for dry gas pressure. Table 4-1 shows gas pressures at several altitudes.

Note that PIO_2 in Table 4-1 refers to air in the trachea. At this point in the airway, water vapor has been added so that water vapor pressure (47 mm Hg) must be subtracted from the barometric pressure to obtain the PIO_2. In Chapter 1 we calculated the PO_2 in dry air and arrived at a figure of 134 mm Hg for Denver; once in the trachea, the PO_2 is 125 mm Hg.

What is the PIO_2 (in the trachea) of a patient breathing ambient air in Cleveland?

?
a) 147 mm Hg
b) 713 mm Hg
c) Must measure barometric pressure

While purists might answer c, the slight day-to-day variation in average barometric pressure is not critical to this calculation. In Cleveland, where average P_B is about 747 mm Hg, the PIO_2 breathing ambient (room) air is

$$.21(747-47) = 147 \text{ mm Hg.}$$

TABLE 4-1. Gas Pressures at Various Altitudes*

LOCATION	ALT.	P_B	FIO_2	PIO_2	$PaCO_2$	PAO_2	PaO_2
Sea Level	0	760	.21	150	40	102	95
Cleveland	500	747	.21	147	40	99	92
Denver	5280	640	.21	125	34	84	77
Pike's Peak	14114	450	.21	85	30	62	55
Mt. Everest	29028	253	.21	43	7.5	35	28

*ALT. = altitude in feet; all pressures in mm Hg
P_B = barometric pressure
FIO_2 = fraction of inspired oxygen
PIO_2 = pressure of inspired oxygen in the trachea
$PaCO_2$ = arterial PCO_2, assumed to = alveolar PCO_2
PAO_2 = alveolar PO_2. PAO_2 is calculated using an assumed
    R value of 0.8 except for the summit of Mt. Everest,
    where 0.85 is used (West 1983)
PaO_2 = arterial PO_2, assuming a $P(A-a)O_2$ of 7 mm Hg at each
    altitude; each PaO_2 value is normal for its respective
    altitude

Do all these assumptions (about P_B, R value, water vapor pressure, etc.) weaken the validity of the alveolar gas equation? Not at all. Assumptions in clinical use of the alveolar gas equation (see Table 4-2) allow PAO_2 to be readily calculated and used for patient assessment. It is always amusing to see someone report an alveolar-arterial PO_2 difference to the decimal point, e.g., 25.7 mm Hg; such precision is not only impossible to obtain, and therefore specious, it is clinically unnecessary.

Table 4-2. Assumptions in Clinical Use of the Alveolar Gas Equation

1. Accurate barometric pressure is known at time blood is drawn
2. Respiratory quotient is 0.8
3. $PaCO_2 = PACO_2$
4. Water vapor pressure is 47 mm Hg
5. Accurate FIO_2 is known when the patient is breathing supplemental oxygen

4.1 What is the tracheal PIO_2 at sea level when the FIO_2 is .40?

a) 100 mm Hg
b) 150 mm Hg
c) 200 mm Hg
d) 285 mm Hg
e) Indeterminate without additional information

4.2 What is the PAO_2 at sea level in the following circumstances?

a) $FIO_2 = 1.00$, $PaCO_2 = 30$ mm Hg
b) $FIO_2 = .21$, $PaCO_2 = 50$ mm Hg
c) $FIO_2 = .40$, $PaCO_2 = 30$ mm Hg

4.3 What is the PAO_2 on the summit of Mt. Everest in the following circumstances?

a) $FIO_2 = .21$, $PaCO_2 = 40$ mm Hg
b) $FIO_2 = 1.00$, $PaCO_2 = 40$ mm Hg
c) $FIO_2 = .21$, $PaCO_2 = 10$ mm Hg

The alveolar-arterial PO_2 difference

By comparing the *calculated* PAO_2 with the *measured* PaO_2, we can learn much useful information about the patient's state of gas exchange. As already pointed out, PaO_2 can never be higher than PAO_2 and should always be lower. The *difference* between the two PO_2 values depends on several factors, particularly the distribution of ventilation to perfusion among the millions of alveolar-capillary units.

It is important to distinguish between *diffusion block* and *ventilation-perfusion imbalance* as physiologic causes of hypoxemia. Both processes affect oxygen transfer from air into blood but only the latter process plays a clinically significant role in hypoxemia.

Diffusion is the physiologic mechanism by which gas moves across a membrane, from a region of higher to one of lower pressure; it describes the movement of oxygen from the individual alveolar spaces across the alveolar-capillary membrane and into the pulmonary capillary blood, and the movement of CO_2 in the opposite direction.

Both oxygen and carbon dioxide diffuse across the alveolar-capillary membrane because of their respective pressure differences between alveolus and capillary blood. Diffusion of either gas is so rapid and efficient that any lung disease manifested by a "diffusion barrier" (e.g., pulmonary fibrosis, congestive heart failure) does not cause significant hypoxemia in patients at rest.

Diffusion block *may* cause hypoxemia under certain circumstances, e.g., exercise in patients with interstitial fibrosis. With CO_2, diffusion impairment is *never* a cause of CO_2 retention under any circumstances. It is a common misconception to attribute CO_2 retention to a diffusion block; patients retain CO_2 because of under-ventilation of alveoli, never because of diffusion impairment.

The term "ventilation-perfusion," abbreviated V-Q, refers to the amount of air entering the alveoli per minute *relative* to the capillary perfusion of those alveoli. A ventilation-perfusion ratio of 1.0 means that an amount of ventilation in an alveolar unit (e.g., 1 ml/min) is available to exchange gases with an equal amount of capillary blood in that unit (1 ml/min). Equality of ventilation to perfusion is the ideal. Figure 4-3 shows the range of V-Q ratios.

"V-Q imbalance" occurs when there is more or less ventilation for the amount of perfusion. For example, if there is twice as much ventilation in an alveolus for the amount of capillary perfusion, the V-Q ratio of that unit is 2.0; if there is half as much ventilation as perfusion, the V-Q ratio is 0.5, etc.

In the normal upright lung, apical alveoli have high V-Q ratios and basilar alveoli have low V-Q ratios. High V-Q ratios result in alveolar dead space (physiologic dead space) and wasted ventilation (see Chapter 3); blood leaving these units has a relatively high PO_2 and low PCO_2. Low V-Q ratios result in under-ventilation and pulmonary capillary blood that is poorly oxygenated, or venous admixture (venous blood is "admixed" with normally oxygenated blood). Compared to the average for the lungs, blood leaving low V-Q units has a relatively low PO_2 and a relatively high PCO_2 (Figure 4-3).

Note that blood coursing through alveolar units with no ventilation constitutes a V-Q ratio of zero for those units; this is colloquially called a "shunt" (technically, a "right-to-left shunt of pulmonary capillary blood"). V-Q units of zero have the same effect on oxygenation as if the blood were shunted anatomically (e.g., through an arterio-venous fistula). A shunt, therefore, is really an extreme of V-Q imbalance. No amount of inhaled oxygen can oxygenate shunted blood, whereas given enough FIO_2 and time, blood perfusing low V-Q units can be oxygenated.

Although the normal lung has both high and low V-Q units, the V-Q ratios tend to balance, so that the *overall* V-Q distribution of the normal lung approaches one. Even so, the over-ventilated units cannot compensate fully for under-oxygenation resulting from the low or zero V-Q units. For this reason the arterial PO_2 ends up slightly lower than the alveolar PO_2. This normal difference between alveolar and arterial PO_2 is due to V-Q inequality and *not* to any diffusion barrier.

Figure 4-3. The range of V-Q ratios. Alveolar-capillary units with low V-Q ratios represent venous admixture. Units with high V-Q ratios represent alveolar dead space. (From Martin L.: Pulmonary Physiology in Clinical Practice, Copyright 1987 by the C.V. Mosby Co., St. Louis.)

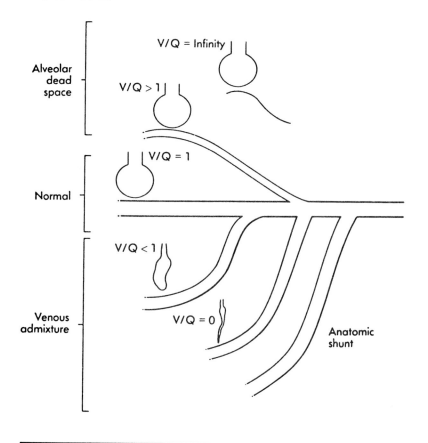

Given a normal V-Q ratio, the PO_2 of blood leaving the alveolus ("end-capillary" PO_2) is almost identical to the alveolar PO_2 (see Figure 4-2). An A-a PO_2 difference arises because some units are under-ventilated for the amount of blood perfusing them; when blood leaving these units mixes with the over-oxygenated blood from high V-Q units, the result is invariably a PO_2 lower than the mean alveolar PO_2. Simply stated, the greater the degree of V-Q imbalance, the worse the hypoxemia. (As long as there is sufficient alveolar ventilation, CO_2 will be unaffected by degrees of V-Q imbalance that routinely lead to hypoxemia).

The term "A-a gradient" is really a misnomer because the difference between mean alveolar PO_2 and arterial PO_2 is due to V-Q imbalance or diffusion impairment, not to any oxygen gradient between alveolus and pulmonary capillary blood. The physiologically correct term is "A-a O_2 difference." This difference — one of oxygen pressures — will be notated here as $P(A-a)O_2$.

?
If there was no V-Q imbalance the $P(A-a)O_2$ would be a) same as with V-Q imbalance or b) almost zero?

If there was no V-Q imbalance, the $P(A-a)O_2$ would be almost zero. The difference between alveolar and end-capillary PO_2 is negligible when ventilation matches perfusion and the alveolar-capillary membrane is of normal thickness; diffusion of oxygen across the membrane is "complete" in normal lungs. A finite $P(A-a)O_2$ exists because V-Q imbalance in healthy lungs (a result mainly of gravity) leads to some low V-Q units, i.e., units with relatively poorer ventilation for the amount of perfusion; this situation occurs mainly in the lung bases.

These low V-Q units result in a reduced end-capillary PO_2; this, in turn, depresses the arterial PO_2 to a level below the mean alveolar PO_2 value. Without any V-Q imbalance (a non-existent ideal) the average of *all* end-capillary PO_2 values — and hence the arterial PO_2 — would equal the mean alveolar PO_2.

The normal range for P(A-a)O$_2$ is:

?
a) 5-15 mm Hg for young to middle-aged people breathing ambient air (FIO$_2$ .21)
b) 15-25 mm Hg for elderly people, FIO$_2$ .21
c) 5-110 mm Hg, when breathing 100% oxygen
d) all of the above

Although normal P(A-a)O$_2$ is sometimes quoted as "5 to 15," that is true only for the conditions specified in answer a. Elderly people have a higher normal P(A-a)O$_2$ (Figure 4-4). Sorbini et al. calculated the relationship (for healthy supine individuals) as PaO$_2$ = 109 - 0.43(age in years). Finally, since P(A-a)O$_2$ varies with FIO$_2$ (Figure 4-5), all choices are correct.

Figure 4-4. Decline of PaO$_2$ and increase in P(A-a)O$_2$ with increasing age. (PaO$_2$ line drawn from data in Sorbini et al., Arterial oxygen tension in healthy subjects, Respiration, 1968).

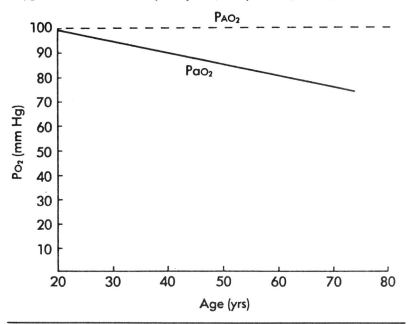

Figure 4-5. Normal range of P(A-a)O₂ from FIO₂ of .21 to 1.00, based on data obtained from 16 healthy subjects age 40 to 50 years (Harris, et al., The normal alveolar-arterial oxygen tension gradient in man, Clin Sci Mol Med 1974). Lines represent mean values + or - 2 standard deviations (SD). P(A-a)O₂ increases with increasing FIO₂ up to 0.6, then reaches a plateau with further increases in FIO₂. Note that the P(A-a)O₂ may normally exceed 100 mm Hg when FIO₂ is 1.00.

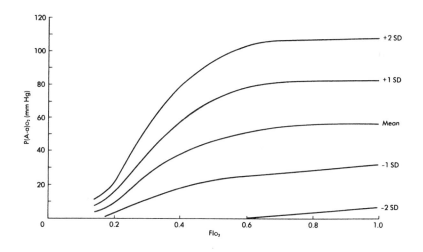

Are the lungs transferring oxygen properly? The clinical usefulness of P(A-a)O₂

If PIO₂ is held constant and PaCO₂ increases, PAO₂ (and PaO₂) will always decrease. Since PAO₂ is a calculation based on known (or assumed) factors, its change is predictable. PaO₂, by contrast, is a measurement with a theoretical maximum value defined by PAO₂ and an actual value determined by the state of ventilation-perfusion imbalance, cardiac output, and O₂ content of blood entering the pulmonary artery (mixed venous blood). In particular, the greater the imbalance of ventilation-perfusion ratios, the more PaO_2 tends to differ from the calculated PAO_2.

CASE.   A 27-year-old young woman came to the emergency department complaining of pleuritic chest pain. She had been taking birth control pills. Her chest x-ray and physical exam were normal. Arterial blood gas showed pH 7.45, $PaCO_2$ 31 mm Hg, HCO_3^- 21 mEq/L, PaO_2 83 mm Hg (FIO_2 .21; P_B 747 mm Hg). Viral pleurodynia was presumptively diagnosed in the patient, who was discharged home with a prescription for pain medication.

What was this patient's PIO_2, PAO_2 and $P(A-a)O_2$ in the emergency room?

?
PIO_2 _____

PAO_2 _____

$P(A-a)O_2$ _____

This young woman's PaO_2 was initially judged normal and her defect in oxygen transfer went unappreciated. The calculated PIO_2 and PAO_2 were 147 and 110 mm Hg, respectively; thus her $P(A-a)O_2$ was elevated at 27 mm Hg (110-83), indicating gas transfer abnormality. She returned the next day with similar complaints; a lung scan was done and interpreted as "high probability" for pulmonary embolism (PE). PE was no doubt the cause of her increased $P(A-a)O_2$ when she was first seen.

As this case illustrates, the principal value of calculating PAO_2 is to allow for proper interpretation of a given PaO_2. Let's say you have a blood gas result showing a PaO_2 of 55 mm Hg. Why is it lower than normal? From low barometric pressure? Low FIO_2? Hypoventilation? Or does the low PaO_2 represent a gas exchange defect within the lungs (and therefore ventilation-perfusion imbalance)?   Answers to these everyday clinical questions can often be obtained by calculating the alveolar PO$_2$ and then the alveolar-arterial PO$_2$ difference.

One cannot properly assess *any* PaO$_2$ without knowing, at minimum, the barometric pressure, FIO$_2$ and PaCO$_2$, information incorporated in the equation for PAO$_2$. Consider the following three PaO$_2$ values: 95 mm Hg, 60 mm Hg, and 28 mm Hg. Based solely on the "normal range" for PaO$_2$, the first value seems normal and the other two reduced, the last one critically so. However, do any of the three values represent a problem with gas exchange? From these values alone could you decide if the lungs are working properly? Could the "normal" PaO$_2$ reflect a serious gas exchange problem? Could there be *no* gas exchange problem with the other two values?

?

Under what circumstance could a PaO$_2$ of 95 mm Hg represent severe gas exchange abnormality?

A PaO$_2$ of 95 mm Hg would be abnormal in anyone breathing 100% oxygen unless the barometric pressure was very low. What should the PaO$_2$ be in a 42-year-old man inhaling pure oxygen? (Assume a normal P(A-a)O$_2$ of 100 mm Hg on this FIO$_2$, normal ventilation and a barometric pressure of 760 mm Hg).

?
a) 100 mm Hg
b) 250 mm Hg
c) over 550 mm Hg

Using the alveolar gas equation we find that

$$PAO_2 = 1.00 \ (760 - 47) - 40 \ mm \ Hg = 673 \ mm \ Hg$$

If his PaO_2 was only 95 mm Hg, $P(A-a)O_2$ would be 578 mm Hg and would signify a critical gas exchange problem and a critical illness, e.g., pulmonary edema or the adult respiratory distress syndrome. Without the additional information provided by the PAO_2 calculation, there is no way to assess whether a PaO_2 of 95 mm Hg reflects normal or abnormal gas exchange.

?

Under what circumstances could a PaO_2 of 60 mm Hg represent no gas exchange abnormality?

Again, you need to know the FIO_2, barometric pressure, and $PaCO_2$; any one of these three factors could reduce PAO_2 without any defect in the gas exchange function of the lungs.

?

What is the $P(A-a)O_2$ of a 35-year-old woman who took an overdose of sleeping pills and has a $PaCO_2$ of 65 mm Hg, PaO_2 60 mm Hg? Assume barometric pressure is 760 mm Hg and the patient is breathing ambient air.

Using the alveolar gas equation we find that

$$PAO_2 = .21 \ (713) - 1.2(65) = 72 \text{ mm Hg}$$

Since PaO_2 is 60 mm Hg, the $P(A-a)O_2$ is 12 mm Hg, a normal value. The patient is globally hypoventilating because of the drug overdose, but she has no problem with exchanging oxygen within her lungs. The normal $P(A-a)O_2$ suggests normal lung function in terms of gas exchange and that the problem (at this point) is hypoventilation from central nervous system depression.

If, under identical circumstances, her PaO_2 was measured at 40 mm Hg, then $P(A-a)O_2$ would be 32 mm Hg and you would want to search for a pulmonary condition such as aspiration pneumonia or pulmonary edema to explain the defect in gas exchange.

?

Under what circumstances could a healthy individual have a PaO_2 of 28 mm Hg?

Again, you have to know the FIO_2, barometric pressure and $PaCO_2$. A very low FIO_2 could explain this PaO_2. A subject breathing an FIO_2 of only 8% would have a PIO_2 of 57 mm Hg at sea level; with hyperventilation, for example to 20 mm Hg, the calculated alveolar PO_2 would be about 33 mm Hg and $P(A-a)O_2$ 5 mm Hg. The problem in such a case is not with pulmonary gas exchange but the environment.

A PaO_2 of 28 mm Hg would also be normal under ambient conditions on the summit of Mt. Everest, where barometric pressure is only 253 mm Hg, PIO_2 only 43 mm Hg (Table 4-1). To survive without supplemental oxygen at the summit (a feat accomplished by several people), the climber has to hyperventilate markedly. If the climber maintained $PaCO_2$ at 40 mm Hg, his PAO_2 would be *minus* 5 mm Hg, a value wholly incompatible with life!

On one expedition to the summit, 10 minutes after supplemental O_2 was removed, a climber's end-tidal PCO_2 (equivalent to $PACO_2$) was measured at 7.5 mm Hg. The calculated PAO_2 was only 35 mm Hg. Based on a theoretic $P(A-a)O_2$ of 7 mm Hg, West and colleagues determined the climber's PaO_2 at the summit to be an astonishing 28 mm Hg — extremely low but "normal" for the circumstances (West 1983).

In summary, to properly interpret PaO_2 one needs to know PAO_2, a calculation based on barometric pressure, FIO_2, water vapor pressure and $PaCO_2$.

4-4. For each of the following case examples, calculate the $P(A-a)O_2$ using the abbreviated alveolar gas equation and a barometric pressure of 760 mm Hg. Which of these patients is most likely to have lung disease? Do any of the values represent a measurement or recording error?

a) A 35-year-old patient with $PaCO_2$ 50 mm Hg, PaO_2 150 mm Hg, FIO_2 .40.

b) A 44-year-old patient with $PaCO_2$ 75 mm Hg, PaO_2 95 mm Hg, FIO_2 0.28.

c) A young, anxious patient with PaO_2 120 mm Hg, $PaCO_2$ 15 mm Hg, FIO_2 0.21.

d) A patient in the intensive care unit with PaO_2 350 mm Hg, $PaCO_2$ 40 mm Hg, FIO_2 0.80.

e) A patient with PaO_2 80 mm Hg, $PaCO_2$ 72 mm Hg, FIO_2 .21.

What is the implication of an elevated $P(A-a)O_2$?

If $P(A-a)O_2$ is elevated above normal, the patient has a defect in gas exchange; some portion of the pulmonary circulation is inadequately oxygenated. Thus the problem can be considered of *pulmonary* origin: an abnormal lung condition interfering with gas exchange. (A relatively rare non-pulmonary cause for increased $P(A-a)O_2$ is right to left intracardiac shunt; this can usually be ruled out by clinical exam and echocardiography.)

The principal causes of a low PaO_2 and/or increased $P(A-a)O_2$ are listed in Table 4-3. Although three non-respiratory and four respiratory causes are listed, significant hypoxemia is almost always due to V-Q imbalance and its variant, right-to-left shunting. Mixed venous blood with a low O_2 content can depress the resulting PaO_2, but even this phenomenon is not significant unless there is severe V-Q imbalance or a right to left shunt.

TABLE 4-3. Physiologic causes of a low PaO$_2$ and elevated P(A-a)O$_2$

Causes	Effect on P(A-a)O$_2$
Non-respiratory	
Cardiac right-to-left shunt	Increased
Decreased PIO$_2$	Normal
Low mixed venous oxygen content	Increased
Respiratory	
Pulmonary right-to-left shunt	Increased
Ventilation-perfusion imbalance	Increased
Diffusion barrier	Increased
Hypoventilation (increased PaCO$_2$)	Normal

Answers to numbered questions

4-1. PIO_2 refers to the tracheal PO_2, so water vapor has to be subtracted from the sea level barometric pressure of 760 mm Hg. The FIO_2 is given as .40. Hence

$$PIO_2 = .40(760 - 47) = 285 \text{ mm Hg.}$$

4-2. To calculate PAO_2 the $PaCO_2$ must be subtracted from the PIO_2. Again, the barometric pressure is 760 mm Hg since the values are obtained at sea level. In part a), the $PaCO_2$ of 30 mm Hg is not multiplied by 1.2 since the FIO_2 is 1.00. In parts b) and c) the factor 1.2 is multiplied times the $PaCO_2$.

a) $PAO_2 = 1.00(713) - 30 = 683 \text{ mm Hg}$

b) $PAO_2 = .21(713) - 1.2(50) = 90 \text{ mm Hg}$

c) $PAO_2 = .40(713) - 1.2(30) = 249 \text{ mm Hg}$

4-3. The PAO_2 on the summit of Mt. Everest is calculated just as at sea level, using the barometric pressure of 253 mm Hg. (Although the respiratory quotient is not known — West and colleagues assumed a value of .85 — you can use the same abbreviated equation as in problem 4-2.)

a) $PAO_2 = .21(253 - 47) - 1.2(40) = - 5 \text{ mm Hg}$

b) $PAO_2 = 1.00(253 - 47) - 40 = 166 \text{ mm Hg}$

c) $PAO_2 = .21(253 - 47) - 1.2(10) = 31 \text{ mm Hg}$

Answers to numbered questions (continued)

4-4.

a) $PAO_2 = .40 (760 - 47) - 1.2(50)$
  $= 225$ mm Hg
  $P(A-a)O_2 = 225 - 150 = 75$ mm Hg

The $P(A-a)O_2$ is elevated but still within the normal range for this FIO_2 (see Figure 4-5), so the patient may or may not have a defect in gas exchange.

b) $PAO_2 = .28(713) - 1.2(75)$
  $= 200 - 90 = 110$ mm Hg
  $P(A-a)O_2 = 110 - 95 = 15$ mm Hg

Despite severe hypoventilation, there is no evidence for lung disease. Hypercapnia is most likely a result of disease involving the central nervous system or chest bellows.

c) $PAO_2 = .21(713) - 1.2(15)$
  $= 150 - 18 = 132$ mm Hg
  $P(A-a)O_2 = 132 - 120 = 12$ mm Hg

Hyperventilation can easily raise PaO_2 above 100 mm Hg when the lungs are normal, as in this case.

d) $PAO_2 = .80 (713) - 40 = 530$ mm Hg

(Note that the factor 1.2 is dropped since FIO_2 is above 60%)

Answers to numbered questions (continued)

4-4.

d) (continued)

$P(A-a)O_2 = 530 - 350 = 180$ mm Hg

Despite very high PaO_2, the lungs are not transferring oxygen normally.

e) $PAO_2 = .21 \ (713) - 1.2(72)$
$= 150 - 86 = 64$ mm Hg
$P(A-a)O_2 = 64 - 80 = -16$ mm Hg

A negative $P(A-a)O_2$ is incompatible with life. This is a not uncommon laboratory result and can be explained by: incorrect FIO_2, incorrect blood gas measurement, or a reporting or transcription error.

CHAPTER 5.

SaO$_2$ and Oxygen Content

How much oxygen is in the blood?

In Chapter 4 you learned how to assess PaO$_2$ as an indicator of gas exchange, by comparing it with the alveolar PO$_2$. You learned that, depending on the PAO$_2$, a PaO$_2$ of 50 mm Hg could reflect no lung problem whatsoever (e.g., at high altitude) while a PaO$_2$ of 90 mm Hg could reflect a severe gas exchange abnormality (if the patient was receiving a high FIO$_2$).

It is also important to know whether the level of oxygen in the blood is adequate. Three different terms are used to describe oxygen levels in the blood: oxygen *pressure*, oxygen *saturation* and oxygen *content*. These terms are defined in the following paragraphs and illustrated schematically in Figure 5-1.

OXYGEN PRESSURE. Oxygen molecules dissolved in plasma (i.e., not bound to hemoglobin) are free to impinge on the measuring electrode; this "impingement" of O$_2$ molecules is reflected as a pressure, the PO$_2$ (in an arterial blood sample, the PaO$_2$). Although the number of O$_2$ molecules dissolved in plasma determines, along with other factors, how many will bind to hemoglobin, once bound the oxygen molecules no longer exert any pressure; bound molecules are no longer free to hit the measuring electrode. Since PaO$_2$ reflects only those oxygen molecules dissolved in plasma and not those bound to hemoglobin, PaO$_2$ does not tell us "how much" oxygen is in the blood; that information is given by the oxygen content.

OXYGEN SATURATION. Binding sites for oxygen are the heme groups, the Fe^{++}-porphyrin portions of the hemoglobin molecule. Heme sites occupied by oxygen molecules are said to be "saturated" with oxygen. The percentage of all the available

Figure 5-1. Oxygen pressure, saturation and content. Schematic shows cross section of an arterial blood vessel. Free oxygen molecules (O_2 with arrows) have motion in plasma that is measured as a pressure (in arterial blood, PaO_2). Each hemoglobin molecule has four $Fe^{++}Heme$ sites for binding O_2. Oxygen-bound molecules ($O_2:Fe^{++}Heme$), in equilibrium with the dissolved O_2 molecules, exert no gaseous pressure. The percentage of $Fe^{++}Heme$ sites bound with oxygen is the "saturation of arterial blood with oxygen" (SaO_2). In this example 30 of 32 $Fe^{++}Heme$ sites are bound with O_2 so the SaO_2 is 93.8%.

The total number of O_2 molecules per aliquot of blood — both unbound (dissolved) and bound — constitutes the oxygen content. Oxygen content in arterial blood is written CaO_2 and has units of ml O_2/dl blood. Normal O_2 content ranges from 16 to 22 ml O_2/dl (depending on the hemoglobin content). Approximately 98% of the normal O_2 content is carried bound to hemoglobin.

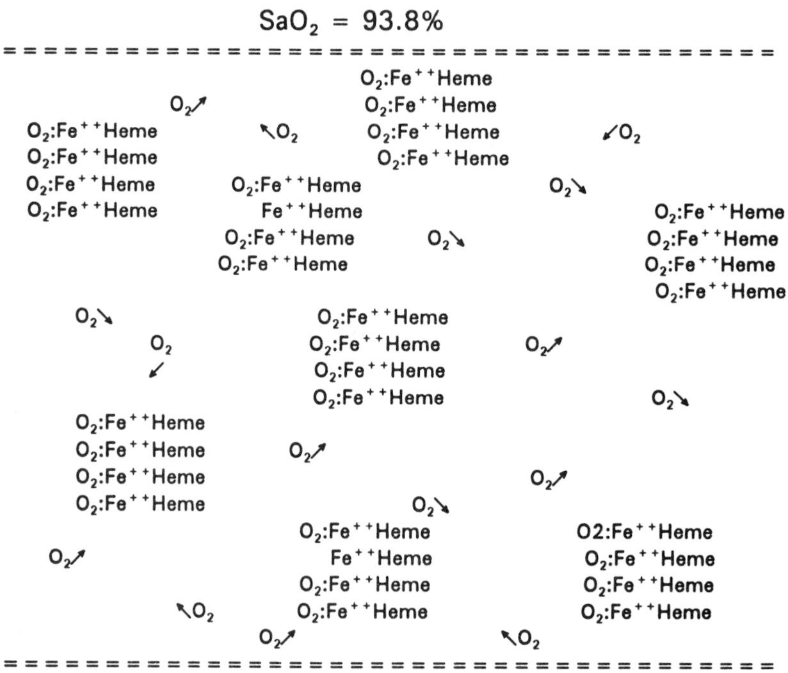

$$SaO_2 = 93.8\%$$

heme binding sites saturated with oxygen is the hemoglobin oxygen saturation (in arterial blood, the SaO_2). In Figure 5-1, 30 of 32 sites are bound with O_2 so the O_2 saturation is 93.8%. Oxygen saturation is determined largely by the PO_2 in the blood but other factors have an influence, such as pH and temperature. Because SaO_2 is a percentage, it can never be higher than 100%.

OXYGEN CONTENT. Tissues need a requisite amount of O_2 molecules for metabolism. Neither the pressure of oxygen in the blood nor the percent saturation of hemoglobin tells us *how much* oxygen is in the blood. *How much* is provided by the oxygen content, with units ml O_2/dl. Oxygen content can be calculated by the oxygen content equation (introduced in Chapter 2):

$$CaO_2 \; = \; (Hb \; x \; 1.34 \; x \; SaO_2) \; + \; (.003 \; x \; PaO_2).$$

As shown by the equation, oxygen content includes oxygen bound to hemoglobin (Hb x 1.34 x SaO_2) *and* oxygen dissolved in plasma (.003 x PaO_2). The amount of oxygen bound to hemoglobin is the product of the hemoglobin content (Hb, in gm/dl), the oxygen carrying capacity of hemoglobin (1.34 ml O_2/gm), and the hemoglobin oxygen saturation (SaO_2). This equation can be used to calculate oxygen content of any blood or plasma sample.

?

Figure 5-2 shows two beakers containing liquid open to the atmosphere. Beaker 1 contains blood with a hemoglobin content of 15 grams%. Beaker 2 contains only plasma (no hemoglobin). Assuming a barometric pressure of 760 mm Hg (and no water vapor pressure), calculate the *oxygen content* in each beaker.

Beaker 1 contains hemoglobin that will combine chemically with oxygen; hence the oxygen content in beaker 1 consists of bound and unbound (dissolved) oxygen molecules. In beaker 2 there is no hemoglobin, just pure plasma; all of its oxygen content must come from dissolved oxygen.

Figure 5-2. Beaker 1 contains blood with a hemoglobin content of 15 grams%; beaker 2 contains pure plasma, no hemoglobin. Both beakers are open to the atmosphere (dry air; barometric pressure 760 mm Hg).

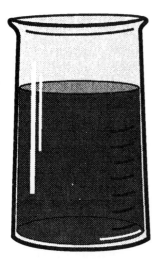 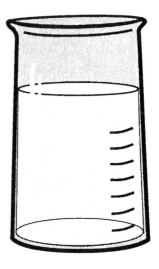

Beaker 1
Blood (15 grams%
hemoglobin)

Beaker 2
Plasma only

Dissolved oxygen in both beakers is determined by the PO_2 to which the liquid is exposed and the solubility of oxygen in plasma. The solubility is .003 ml O_2/dl plasma/mm Hg. But what is the PO_2? Because there is no CO_2 exchange taking place in either beaker (as there is in our lungs) and the surface of the liquid is in free contact with the atmosphere, the PO_2 *in* solution is simply the PO_2 *above* the solution. Given a barometric pressure of 760 mm Hg (dry air), the PO_2 in both beakers is

$$FIO_2 \times P_B = .21 \times 760 \text{ mm Hg} = 160 \text{ mm Hg.}$$

Since the PO_2 is equal in both beakers, the O_2 content represented by *dissolved oxygen* is also the same in both beakers; this content is

?
a)   .48 ml O_2/dl
b)   2.0 ml O_2/dl
c)   4.8 ml O_2/dl

To calculate content from dissolved oxygen, substitute the values for oxygen solubility and PO_2:

O_2 content of dissolved O_2 = .003 ml O_2/dl/mm Hg x 160 mm Hg

$\qquad$ = .48 ml O_2/dl

There is no hemoglobin in beaker 2 so the *entirety* of its O_2 content comes from dissolved oxygen and = .48 ml O_2/dl. There is far more oxygen content in beaker 1 because oxygen molecules combine chemically with hemoglobin.   Once combined, O_2 molecules no longer exert any pressure. As O_2 molecules are taken up by hemoglobin, additional molecules enter the plasma portion of the blood from the atmosphere. (Hemoglobin is like a giant sponge that soaks up oxygen molecules and allows many more to enter the surrounding plasma.) Thus the difference in oxygen content between the two beakers is the amount of oxygen bound to hemoglobin.

The oxygen content represented by *hemoglobin-bound* oxygen in beaker 1 is

?
a) .48 ml O_2/dl
b) 15 ml O_2/dl
c) 19.9 ml O_2/dl

O$_2$ content is calculated by the oxygen content equation, which in turn requires knowledge of the O$_2$ saturation of hemoglobin, SaO$_2$. SaO$_2$ is determined by the PO$_2$ to which the blood is exposed (in this case 160 mm Hg) and the position of the oxygen dissociation curve. With a normally-positioned curve, the SaO$_2$ at this level of PO$_2$ is approximately 99%. (If the relationship of PO$_2$ to SaO$_2$ is not readily apparent to you now, it will be by the end of this chapter.) Thus,

$$
\begin{aligned}
\text{Oxygen content (Hb-bound)} \ &= \ \text{Hb x 1.34 x SaO}_2 \\
&= \ 15 \text{ x } 1.34 \text{ x } .99 \\
&= \ 19.9 \text{ ml O}_2/\text{dl}
\end{aligned}
$$

?
What is the *total* oxygen content of beaker 1? By what factor is this content greater than that in beaker 2?

The total oxygen content of beaker 1 is of course the sum of the dissolved and bound fractions, or .48 + 19.9 = 20.38 ml O$_2$/dl. The total oxygen content of beaker 2 (.48 ml O$_2$/dl) is thus only about 2.4% of that contained in beaker 1. Put another way, beaker 1 contains about *42 times* more oxygen than beaker 2.

?
A healthy man is in the same room as the two beakers. If his PaO$_2$ = 100 mm Hg and hemoglobin content = 15 gms%, what percent of his oxygen content is carried in dissolved form?

The calculation is the same as with the two beakers, except that PO$_2$ is 100 mm Hg instead of 160 mm Hg (PO$_2$ is lower than atmospheric pressure because of the addition of water vapor pressure and PaCO$_2$); thus his dissolved fraction is .3 ml O$_2$/dl instead of .48 ml O$_2$/dl in the beakers. His O$_2$-bound fraction is also slightly lower because a PO$_2$ of 100 mm Hg gives an SaO$_2$ of about 98%. Thus the oxygen content in human blood under these conditions is:

$$
\begin{aligned}
\text{CaO}_2 &= \quad (\text{Hb x } 1.34 \text{ x SaO}_2) \quad + \quad (.003 \text{ x PaO}_2) \\
&= \quad (15 \text{ x } 1.34 \text{ x } .98) \quad + \quad (.003 \text{ x } 100) \\
&= \quad 19.7 \quad\quad\quad\quad\quad + \quad .3 \\
&= \quad 20.0 \text{ ml O}_2/\text{dl}
\end{aligned}
$$

The dissolved O$_2$ content is .3/20 = 1.5% of the total oxygen content. Stated another way, under these conditions (normal PaO$_2$ and hemoglobin content), hemoglobin carries about *67 times more* oxygen than is carried dissolved in the plasma. Clearly, hemoglobin is vital. Under conditions of ambient air and pressure, the content of dissolved oxygen is far too little to meet our metabolic needs.

Although almost all of the oxygen content is chemically bound to hemoglobin, this quantity is unrevealed by knowing only the PaO$_2$. Without knowledge of the hemoglobin content PaO$_2$ does not even give a hint of the total oxygen content. We need to calculate CaO$_2$ to know the *amount* of oxygen in the blood. Because the body needs a requisite oxygen content for survival, and PaO$_2$ alone does not indicate oxygen content, *a patient can have normal or high PaO$_2$ and be starved for oxygen.*

5.1 Which patient is more hypoxemic?

Patient A: PaO$_2$ 85 mm Hg, SaO$_2$ 95%, Hb 7 gm%
Patient B: PaO$_2$ 55 mm Hg, SaO$_2$ 85%, Hb 15 gm%

PaO$_2$ is the most important (but not the only) determinant of SaO$_2$. Think of PaO$_2$ as the driving pressure for oxygen molecules reaching and chemically binding to hemoglobin; the higher the PaO$_2$, the higher the SaO$_2$. The relationship between PaO$_2$ and SaO$_2$ is not linear but "sigmoid-shaped". The relationship is shown by the familiar oxygen dissociation curve (Figure 5-3). The curve is determined from *in vitro* titration of blood with increasing partial pressures of oxygen. At low oxygen pressures there is relatively little increase in SaO$_2$ for a change in PaO$_2$. Above PaO$_2$ of 20 mm Hg, the rate of change of SaO$_2$ increases markedly, then slows again beyond a PaO$_2$ of 60 mm Hg.

The so-called "steep part" of the O_2 dissociation curve is between 20 and 60 mm Hg PaO_2. Compared with the flatter portions, small increases in PaO_2 in this region have a much greater effect on improving SaO_2 and therefore O_2 content. Figure 5-3 also plots PaO_2 against oxygen content for two hemoglobin concentrations, 15 and 10 gm%. Note that the *shape and position* of the curve are the same irrespective of the hemoglobin content.

5.2   Using Figure 5-3, calculate O_2 content of a patient with hemoglobin 12 gms%, PaO_2 50 mm Hg, pH 7.40.

Figure 5-3.   The oxygen dissociation curve. PaO_2 vs. SaO_2 and PaO_2 vs. oxygen content for two hemoglobin values. P_{50} is the PaO_2 at which hemoglobin is 50% saturated with oxygen; normal value is 27 mm Hg. (X represents blood gas values of a case presented later in this chapter). (From Martin L.: Pulmonary Physiology in Clinical Practice, Copyright 1987 by the C.V. Mosby Co., St. Louis.)

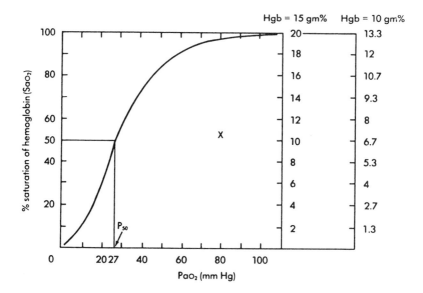

Hypoxemia vs. hypoxia

Question 5-1 asks which patient is more hypoxemic and the answer is found by calculating the oxygen contents. Would the answer have been different if the question was "Which patient is more *hypoxic*?" What is the difference between "hypoxemia" and "hypoxia" and does it matter? Some textbooks use the words interchangeably, whereas others define them differently.

There is no universal agreement on the terms and the distinction is partly semantic. I prefer to define hypoxemia as a reduction in PaO_2, SaO_2 or hemoglobin content (Table 5-1), with the *amount* of oxygen in the blood (oxygen content) as the major determinant of clinical severity. In this context, the lower the oxygen content the more hypoxemic the patient, irrespective of the PaO_2 or SaO_2.

Hypoxia, on the other hand, is a more general term referring to impaired oxygen delivery to the tissues. Hypoxia takes into account cardiac output and oxygen uptake at the tissue level. In this scheme hypoxemia is but one type of hypoxia (Table 5-1). A patient can be hypoxemic but have adequate O_2 delivery to the tissues, through adaptive increases in cardiac output and/or O_2 extraction at the tissue level. Conversely, a patient can have an adequate oxygen content but be hypoxic, as may occur in a low cardiac output state or from mitochondrial oxygen poisoning.

In the final analysis, it doesn't really matter how the terms are used as long as you understand the differences between oxygen pressure, saturation and content. Understand these concepts and you can define hypoxemia and hypoxia any way you wish.

Clinical assessment of hypoxemia

Before the era of rapid blood gas analysis, clinicians would often assess hypoxemia on clinical grounds alone, principally by looking for cyanosis. We now know that clinical assessment of hypoxemia is unreliable (notoriously so), for several reasons:

Table 5-1.   Causes of hypoxia — a general classification

1. Hypoxemia
   a. reduced PaO_2
      (see Table 4-3)
   b. reduced SaO_2
      (any cause of 1a; also, carbon monoxide intoxication, methemoglobinemia, any cause of a right-shifted oxygen dissociation curve, such as acidemia)
   c. reduced hemoglobin content
      (anemia)

2. Reduced oxygen delivery to the tissues
   a. reduced cardiac output
      (shock, congestive heart failure)
   b. left to right systemic shunt
      (e.g., as may be seen in septic shock)

3. Decreased tissue oxygen uptake
   a. mitochondrial poisoning
      (e.g., cyanide poisoning)
   b. left-shifted hemoglobin dissociation curve
      (e.g., alkalemia, carbon monoxide poisoning, abnormal hemoglobin structure)

- There is significant inter-observer variation in detecting cyanosis; some physicians diagnose cyanosis when it cannot be present (normal blood gases) and some miss cyanosis when it is present (very low oxygen saturation) (Comroe 1947).

- It takes approximately 5 gms% of unoxygenated hemoglobin in the capillaries to generate the dark blue color appreciated clinically as cyanosis (Lundsgaard

1923, Martin 1990). Anemic patients may be significantly hypoxemic yet be unable to generate this much reduced hemoglobin. A severely anemic patient whose hemoglobin content was only 5 gms% (giving an hematocrit about 15%) would never manifest cyanosis no matter how hypoxemic.

- Ancillary signs and symptoms of hypoxemia (tachycardia, tachypnea, mental status changes) are so non-specific as to be of no value in reliably detecting hypoxemia. Patients may be profoundly dyspneic with normal PaO_2 and SaO_2. Also, some patients who are profoundly hypoxemic may remain lucid and fully conversant.

If you have any reason to suspect hypoxemia, obtain some measurement of the oxygen level (arterial blood gas or pulse oximetry). There is no clinical substitute for measurement of PaO_2 or SaO_2 when diagnosing hypoxemia or assessing the need for supplemental oxygen therapy.

Oxygenated and reduced hemoglobin

Hypoxemia and hypoxia are not the only terms that often confuse people. Other important terms that need definition and clarification are discussed in this section. Below are arterial blood gas values obtained from a patient breathing room air:

pH	7.42
$PaCO_2$	34 mm Hg
PaO_2	67 mm Hg
SaO_2	84%
%COHb	5%
%MetHb	2%

What are the approximate percentages for each of the following in this patient's blood?

?

oxygenated hemoglobin_____

reducedhemoglobin_____

de-oxygenated hemoglobin_____

oxidized hemoglobin_____

carboxyhemoglobin_____

methemoglobin_____

Oxygenated hemoglobin refers to those heme groups bound with oxygen; it is characterized by the SaO_2 and CaO_2. *Reduced* hemoglobin is another term for *de-oxygenated* hemoglobin and refers to those heme groups unbound to oxygen or to anything else. (Strictly speaking, the terms should be 'oxygenated heme' and 'unoxygenated heme,' since the *same* hemoglobin molecule — with four heme binding sites — could contain *both* oxygenated and unoxygenated heme.)

In the previous blood sample the percentage of oxygenated hemoglobin is the same as the SaO_2, i.e., 84%. The percentage of de-oxygenated (reduced) hemoglobin is found by subtracting all the hemoglobin either bound to something or that cannot bind oxygen; thus the percentage of de-oxygenated hemoglobin is 9%.

Maximum oxygen saturation:	100 %
SaO_2	- 84 %
COHb	- 5 %
MetHb	- 2 %

De-oxygenated hemoglobin:	9 %

Oxidized hemoglobin is hemoglobin with iron in an oxidized state (Fe^{+++}) as opposed to the normal ferrous (Fe^{++}) state; hemoglobin with iron in this state is called *methemoglobin*, in this example given as 2%. Note that even though Fe^{+++} hemoglobin is oxidized, the normal Fe^{++} state of hemoglobin is *not* called "reduced"; reduced hemoglobin refers only to Fe^{++} hemoglobin that is not bound with oxygen or anything else. The terminology is unfortunate but, since it is widely used, you should familiarize yourself with the generally accepted definitions.

Finally, *carboxyhemoglobin* has already been defined, and is given in the problem as 5% of the total hemoglobin.

The importance of measuring (and not just calculating) SaO_2

PaO_2 is a measurement of pressure exerted by oxygen molecules dissolved in plasma; once oxygen molecules chemically bind to hemoglobin, they no longer exert any pressure. Patients can have a reduced PaO_2 (defect in gas transfer) and still have adequate arterial oxygen content, e.g., hemoglobin 15 gms%, PaO_2 55 mm Hg, SaO_2 88%, CaO_2 17.8 ml O_2/dl blood. Conversely, patients can have normal PaO_2 and be *profoundly hypoxemic* from reduced CaO_2. This paradox — normal PaO_2 and hypoxemia — generally occurs two ways: 1) anemia, or 2) altered affinity of hemoglobin for binding oxygen.

> CASE: A 54-year-old man came to the emergency room (ER) complaining of headaches and dyspnea. An arterial blood gas (on room air) showed PaO_2 89 mm Hg, $PaCO_2$ 38 mm Hg, and pH 7.43. SaO_2 was not directly measured but was calculated at 98% based on the measured PaO_2 and a standard oxygen dissociation curve. The patient's hematocrit was 44%. He was sent home after some improvement in the ER and scheduled for a brain CT scan three days later.
>
> The patient was brought back to the ER unconscious the next evening. Ambulance attendants alerted the emergency physicians to a possible faulty heater in the patient's house. This time carbon monoxide and SaO_2 were measured along with routine arterial blood gases.

The results: PaO$_2$ 79 mm Hg, PaCO$_2$ 31 mm Hg, pH 7.36, SaO$_2$ 53%, and carboxyhemoglobin 46%.

What do you suppose was the patient's true SaO$_2$ on the first ER visit?

?
a) probably over 90%
b) probably less than 90%
c) don't know how to guess the answer

The true SaO$_2$ was much lower than 90%, as would have been apparent had it been measured on the first ER visit, instead of just calculated. Generally a patient needs at least 10% COHb to manifest symptoms from excess CO (Table 5-2).

Carbon monoxide per se does not affect PaO$_2$ but only SaO$_2$ and O$_2$ content. (Slight reduction in PaO$_2$ on the second visit was attributed to some basilar atelectasis.) The patient's oxygen saturation and content on the second visit are shown by an "X" in Figure 5-3.

This case illustrates the importance of *measuring* the SaO$_2$ as part of each arterial blood gas test. A *calculated* SaO$_2$ (as shown above) can be misleading. The physician on the first visit missed hypoxemia as a cause of headache and dyspnea because of the falsely "normal" SaO$_2$.

Pulse oximetry

In the last few years pulse oximetry has become widely available as a quick and reliable non-invasive method for measuring SaO$_2$. Because the SaO$_2$ measured by pulse oximetry is not always the same as that measured by CO-oximetry, some authors use the term "SpO$_2$" for the pulse oximetry value. Whatever term is used, knowing the differences should help you avoid the following potential pitfalls when interpreting oxygen saturation obtained by pulse oximetry.

Table 5-2. Symptoms from CO poisoning

% of CO in inspired air	%COHb in blood	Occurrence; signs and symptoms
0	1-2	normal amount from breakdown of heme; no symptoms
< .007	3-10	common in cigarette smokers; no symptoms but may aggravate dyspnea from other causes
.007	>10	found in heavy cigarette and cigar smokers; dyspnea during vigorous exertion; occasional tightness in forehead
.012	>20	dyspnea during moderate exertion; occasional throbbing headache in temples
.022	>30	severe headache; irritability; easy fatigability; disturbed judgment; possible dizziness and possible dimness of vision
.035-.052	>40	headache; confusion; syncope with exertion
.080-.122	>60	unconsciousness; shock; intermittent convulsions; respiratory failure; death if exposure is prolonged
.195	>70	death

1) *Pulse oximetry does not differentiate carboxyhemoglobin from oxyhemoglobin.*   Pulse oximeters are good at separating oxyhemoglobin from reduced (de-oxygenated) hemoglobin by virtue of the two molecules' different absorptions of light.   Carboxyhemoglobin, with a red coloration, absorbs light at a wavelength similar to oxyhemoglobin, so the pulse oximeter reads COHb as oxyhemoglobin. For example, a patient with a true SaO_2 of 85%, plus 10% COHb, will have a pulse oximetry SpO_2 reading of 95%.

2) *Pulse oximetry does not distinguish between oxygen desaturation from a low PaO_2 and from methemoglobin (metHb).* Unlike carbon monoxide, metHb does depress the SpO_2 reading, but not linearly (Barker 1989). MetHb decreases SpO_2 until an SpO_2 of about 85% is reached, at which point SpO_2 stays in the low- to mid-80s with further increases in metHb (Watcha 1989, Ralston 1991). Thus a pulse oximetry SpO_2 of 85% could represent: a) 15% normal de-oxygenated hemoglobin (Fe^{++} unbound with oxygen), a reflection of low PaO_2; b) 15% methemoglobin; *or,* c) some combination of normal oxygen desaturation and excess methemoglobin.

3) *Pulse oximeters tend to give a falsely high reading when the true SaO_2 is very low*, e.g., < 80%. Low SpO_2 values should be confirmed by arterial blood gas measurement of PaO_2 and SaO_2.

4) *Pulse oximetry monitoring may give a false sense of security* if the patient has adequate oxygen saturation but a falling PaO_2 or rising $PaCO_2$. PaO_2 or $PaCO_2$ may change significantly before there is any appreciable change in the SpO_2.

5) *Pulse oximetry may be unreliable if there is poor tissue perfusion.* This problem is most often seen in patients with decreased vascular flow to the extremities.   The

machines only work if there is a strong pulse. With a weak pulse, the SpO_2 reading may "stick" on a false value.

Pulse oximetry is most useful in following a patient's SpO_2 over time (continuous reading), particularly when the oximetry SpO_2 has been correlated with at least one direct measurement of SaO_2. In this setting pulse oximetry can often obviate the need for frequent blood gas monitoring. Conversely, pulse oximetry can often alert one to the need for blood gas measurement, for example, when the SpO_2 reading is lower than expected in a patient receiving supplemental O_2 (Eisenkraft 1988).

?

A 55-year-old man has been hospitalized for three days, following a heart attack. On room air, his pulse oximetry SpO_2 is 85%. His lungs are clear on exam and chest x-ray is normal. Admission arterial blood gas data three days earlier (also obtained on room air) showed a PaO_2 of 84 mm Hg, SaO_2 95%. How would you explain his change in oxygen saturation?

The pulse oximeter SpO_2 could be low because of a low PaO_2, but there was no reason to suspect this; his pulmonary status had not changed over the preceding few days. However, his medications included a long-acting nitrate for coronary artery disease. After the unexpectedly low SpO_2 was found, an arterial blood gas was obtained. PaO_2 was normal at 85 mm Hg, but a low SaO_2 of 84% was confirmed and methemoglobin was measured at 7.2%. The excess methemoglobin was attributed to the nitrate, a known side effect. Without methemoglobin his true oxygen saturation would have been about 92%. The nitrate was discontinued and two days later his pulse oximetry SpO_2 was 92%.

P_{50} and shifts of the oxygen dissociation curve

Many factors can affect the degree of oxygen saturation for a given PaO_2; their net result is the exact shape and position of the oxygen dissociation curve. From the following list choose those factors that affect the binding of oxygen to hemoglobin for a given PaO_2.

?
a)   age of the patient
b) PAO_2
c) $PaCO_2$
d)   pH
e)   carbon monoxide
f)   nature of the hemoglobin molecule
g)   body temperature
h)   2,3-diphosphoglycerate in blood
i)   hemoglobin content

The shape/position of the oxygen dissociation curve depends on all the factors listed above except age of the patient, PAO_2 and hemoglobin content. What about these exceptions?

• Characteristics of the patient (age, body weight, body position, etc.) can affect the PaO_2 by altering ventilation-perfusion relationships (see Chapter 4) but have no direct effect on how oxygen, once in the blood, binds with hemoglobin.

• Although PAO_2 is a major determinant of PaO_2 (see Chapter 4), it has no effect on the binding of oxygen to hemoglobin (i.e., on the SaO_2).

• A common misconception is that anemia somehow changes the binding of oxygen to hemoglobin. In fact, anemia does not affect the position of the O_2 dissociation curve. Stated another way, the amount of hemoglobin affects the O_2 content but not the extent to which oxygen binds to hemoglobin.

All the other listed factors can affect the degree of O_2 binding to hemoglobin for a given PaO_2: $PaCO_2$, pH, carbon monoxide, nature of the hemoglobin molecule, body temperature and 2,3-diphosphoglycerate. Table 5-3 separates these factors according to how they shift the oxygen dissociation curve. Figure 5-4 shows how the curve shifts with changes in pH and temperature.

TABLE 5-3. Conditions that shift the oxygen dissociation curve

<--- To the left	To the right --->

Below normal:
   temperature
   2,3-DPG
   $PaCO_2$
	Above normal:
	   temperature
	   2,3-DPG
	   $PaCO_2$

Elevated:
   COHb, pH
   methemoglobin
	Reduced: pH

Various abnormal hemoglobin chains	Various abnormal hemoglobin chains

A shift of the O_2 dissociation curve to the right means:

?
a) less SaO_2 for a given PaO_2
b) more SaO_2 for a given PaO_2

If a PaO_2 of 60 mm Hg normally gives an SaO_2 of 90%, and the oxygen dissociation curve is shifted to the right, the same PaO_2 will give a lower SaO_2. The correct answer is therefore a.

Figure 5-4. Shifts of the O_2 dissociation curve with changes in pH (top graph; temperature constant) and temperature (bottom graph; pH constant).   (From Slonim NB and Hamilton LH: Respiratory Physiology, 4th ed., Copyright 1981 by the C.V. Mosby Co., St. Louis.)

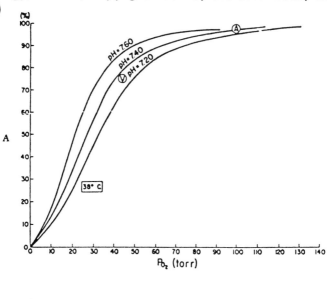

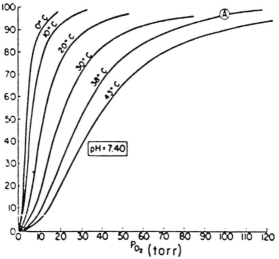

5.3 For the following paired samples, state whether patient (1) or (2) has the lower arterial oxygen content (i.e., which patient is more hypoxemic?).

a) (1) Hb 10 gms%, PaO_2 60 mm Hg, pH 7.55
   (2) Hb 10 gms%, PaO_2 60 mm Hg, pH 7.35

b) (1) Hb 15 gms%, PaO_2 90 mm Hg, pH 7.10
   (2) Hb 15 gms%, PaO_2 60 mm Hg, pH 7.47

c) (1) Hb 12 gms%, SaO_2 90%, pH 7.20
   (2) Hb 12 gms%, SaO_2 80%, pH 7.40

d) (1) Hb 12 gms%, PaO_2 90 mm Hg, pH 7.40
   (2) Hb 12 gms%, SaO_2 90%, pH 7.40

P_{50} is the PaO_2 at which 50% of the arterial hemoglobin is saturated with oxygen, i.e., the PaO_2 at which $SaO_2 = 50\%$. P_{50} is a time-consuming and non-routine measurement, performed only in some blood gas labs on special request. It is used to characterize the degree of shift of the oxygen dissociation curve. Normal P_{50} is about 27 mm Hg.

A rightward shift of the dissociation curve would manifest as:

?
a) P_{50} > 27 mm Hg
b) P_{50} < 27 mm Hg

In which direction is the O_2 dissociation curve shifted if P_{50} is 24 mm Hg?

?
a) to the right
b) to the left

Examination of the oxygen dissociation curve shows that a higher than normal P_{50} reflects a rightward shift of the curve, a lower than normal P_{50} a leftward shift (remember the mnemonic *l*ower, *l*eft).

?

What is better for the hypoxemic patient: left shift or right shift of the curve? Should therapy be directed toward artificially shifting the curve one way or the other? Before answering these questions, study Table 5-4.

Generally, a left-shifted curve results in holding back more oxygen at the tissue level than is gained in the pulmonary capillaries; this results in a paradoxically higher SaO_2 while, at the same time, less oxygen is delivered to the tissues. When the curve is right-shifted the opposite occurs; less oxygen is taken up in the pulmonary capillaries but relatively more is "unloaded" at the tissue level. Some could argue that a right-shifted curve is "better" for the critically ill patient than even a normal dissociation curve. The acidosis accompanying a shock state could be nature's way of delivering more oxygen to the victim.

Unfortunately this physiologic argument doesn't translate into clinical strategy. While a right-shifted curve unloads more oxygen to the tissues, if the shift occurs at the cost of acidemia, high $PaCO_2$ or fever, the patient might suffer in other ways. The best clinical answer to this question is that *neither* shift is better. One should aim for an adequate oxygen content and normal pH and not attempt to manipulate the oxygen dissociation curve.

Carbon Monoxide Poisoning

Figure 5-5 shows how elevated carbon monoxide affects the oxygen dissociation curve. Carbon monoxide affects tissue oxygen delivery in two ways: 1) it reduces arterial oxygen saturation by preventing oxygen binding to hemoglobin; and 2) it increases affinity for those oxygen molecules that do bind to hemoglobin, i.e., it causes a left shift of the oxygen dissociation curve.

Table 5-4. Changes in oxygen content and availability with shifts of the O₂-dissociation curve

	Left-shift	Right shift
Oxygen content in the pulmonary capillaries (site of oxygen uptake)	INCREASED	DECREASED
Oxygen content in the tissue capillaries	INCREASED	DECREASED
Oxygen content released to tissues	DECREASED	INCREASED

Carbon monoxide is about 230 times more avid for hemoglobin than oxygen is. Thus a partial pressure of CO only 1/230 that of oxygen will compete equally for hemoglobin binding sites. If PaO_2 is 100 mm Hg and PaCO is only .43 mm Hg the blood will contain 50% oxyhemoglobin and 50% COHb. Obviously, it only takes tiny amounts of CO to induce poisoning.

Examination of Figure 5-5 shows the "double whammy" effect of excess CO on oxygenation. First, to the extent that CO is bound to hemoglobin, oxygen is prevented from binding to those same sites. Binding of oxygen and CO takes place in the pulmonary capillaries as the gases are inhaled. If enough CO is inhaled to bind with 30% of the hemoglobin (30% COHb), for example, then 30% of the hemoglobin binding sites are effectively prevented from combining with oxygen. The maximum SaO_2 could ever reach is 70%, irrespective of the PaO_2.

Second, CO increases the affinity of hemoglobin for oxygen molecules that *are* chemically bound. Increased affinity means hemoglobin binds oxygen molecules *more tightly* in the presence of excess CO and the oxygen dissociation curve is shifted to the *left*. The adverse effect of this left shift is greatest at the tissue capillary level, as can be seen in Figure 5-5. At PO_2 values found in the tissue capillaries (20 to 40 mm Hg), oxygen is bound more tightly to the hemoglobin, i.e., less is given up to the tissues.

Figure 5-5. Effects of carbon monoxide on oxygen dissociation curve. (Redrawn from Roughton, FJW and Darling, RC: Amer J Physiol 141:17-31;1944 and reproduced with permission from Comroe, JH, Jr: Physiology of Respiration, 2nd ed., Copyright 1974 by Year Book Medical Publishers, Inc., Chicago.)

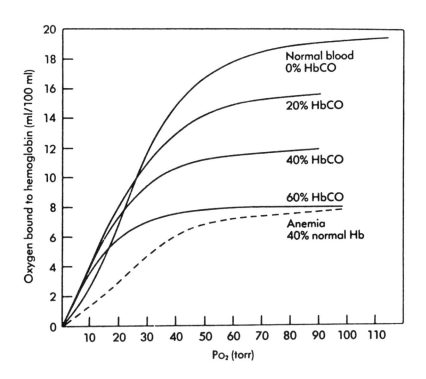

From Figure 5-5 we see that, in the pulmonary capillary, severe anemia (40% of the normal hemoglobin content) has the same effect on O_2 content as 60% COHb. However, when the blood circulates to the tissues, the anemic blood unloads oxygen much more readily than the blood with excess CO. Thus for a given PO_2 at the tissue level (e.g., 30 mm Hg), the oxygen saturation (and content) are much higher in the presence of excess CO; the patient with excess CO is thus more *hypoxic* because the tissues are deprived of oxygen more than from anemia.

In summary, excess CO causes:

● less oxygen to bind to hemoglobin in the pulmonary capillaries.

● oxygen that is taken up by hemoglobin to be held more tightly than normal, making less available to the tissues for any given PO_2 value.

These two effects, plus its very high affinity for hemoglobin, make CO a potent poison.

5-4. Below are blood gas results from four pairs of patients. For each letter pair, state which patient, (1) or (2), is more hypoxemic. Units for hemoglobin content (Hb) are gm% and for PaO_2 mm Hg.

a) (1) Hb 15, PaO_2 100, pH 7.40, COHb 20%
    (2) Hb 12, PaO_2 100, pH 7.40, COHb zero

b) (1) Hb 15, PaO_2 90, pH 7.20, COHb 5%
    (2) Hb 15, PaO_2 50, pH 7.40, COHb 0

c) (1) Hb 5, PaO_2 60, pH 7.40, COHb 0.
    (2) Hb 15, PaO_2 100, pH 7.40, COHb 20%

d) (1) Hb 10, PaO_2 60, pH 7.30, COHb 10%
    (2) Hb 15, PaO_2 100, pH 7.40, COHb 15%

Carbon monoxide is competitively bound to hemoglobin and therefore easily removable if the PO_2 is high enough. Treatment of CO poisoning requires elevating PaO_2 as quickly as possible, the higher the better. In most cases this is accomplished with an FIO_2 equal or close to 100%, for at least the first few hours of therapy. Extreme cases of CO poisoning (presenting with coma or convulsions) require intubation and artificial ventilation with 100% oxygen. In hospitals with a hyperbaric chamber, oxygen can be delivered under increased pressures (e.g., two to three times normal atmospheric pressure), effecting a quicker removal of the CO. The goal in all cases is to "flush out" the CO as quickly as possible with supplemental oxygen.

5-5. A patient comes to the emergency department without assistance, complaining of dyspnea and headaches. Pulse oximetry reading shows an SpO_2 of 94%. How much excess CO could be in this patient's blood?

5-6. A patient comatose from CO poisoning is brought to the hospital. Initial arterial blood gas on room air reveals pH 7.30, $PaCO_2$ 30 mm Hg, PaO_2 85 mm Hg, SaO_2 45%, COHb 52%, and hemoglobin content 15 gm%. Calculate the patient's arterial PO_2 and oxygen content under each of the conditions listed below. In each situation, assume no change in $PaCO_2$; a uniform $P(A-a)O_2$ of 50 mm Hg; and a sea level elevation for the hospital.

a) 80% oxygen by face mask, CO level down to 45%.

b) Intubated, on 100% FIO_2, CO level down to 40%.

c) In a hyperbaric chamber at two atmospheres pressure (=1520 mm Hg), on 100% FIO_2, CO level down to 40%.

d) In a hyperbaric chamber at three atmospheres pressure (=2280 mm Hg), on 50% oxygen, CO level down to 30%.

5-7.   With 100% inspired oxygen, approximately how many atmospheres of pressure are necessary to provide an arterial oxygen content in the plasma phase that would equal the total arterial content available when breathing room air at sea level? Calculate your answer for a patient with normal lungs and hemoglobin content.

  a) 4
  b) 6
  c) 9
  d) 15
  e) 20

5-8.   A patient with no history of respiratory disease has endoscopy for a stomach problem. He is given 3 L/min nasal O_2 and SpO_2 is monitored with a pulse oximeter. At the beginning of the procedure SpO_2 is 99%; halfway through endoscopy SpO_2 is noted to be 91%. The patient shows no respiratory distress. What is your explanation for the change in SpO_2? What should be done?

Answers to numbered questions

5-1.   The body needs oxygen molecules, so oxygen content (CaO_2) takes precedence over partial pressure in determining degrees of hypoxemia. In this problem the amount of oxygen contributed by the dissolved fraction is negligible and will not affect the answer.

Patient A
$CaO_2 = .95 \times 7 \times 1.34 = 8.9$ ml O_2/dl

Patient B
$CaO_2 = .85 \times 15 \times 1.34 = 17.1$ ml O_2/dl

Patient A, with the higher PaO_2, is more hypoxemic.

5-2.   Hemoglobin 12 gms%, PaO_2 50 mm Hg, pH 7.40. To calculate oxygen content, you first need to find the SaO_2. From Figure 5-3, you can see that SaO_2 is about 83% (in using the graph +/- 1% is acceptable). Ignoring the dissolved oxygen fraction (which is very small), the O_2 content is

$$CaO_2 = .83 \times 12 \times 1.34 = 13.35 \text{ ml } O_2/\text{dl}$$

Note that this content falls midway between the oxygen content values for hemoglobin of 10 and 15 gms%.

5-3.   For these comparisons you needed to check Figure 5-4 for the SaO_2 values for the given pH and PaO_2. (Expect some slight variation in SaO_2 values from those shown below.) The amount of oxygen contributed by the dissolved fraction is negligible and will not affect the answer.

(continued)

Answers to numbered questions (continued)

5-3. (continued)

    a) (1) CaO_2 = .93 x 10 x 1.34 = 12.5 ml O_2/dl
       (2) CaO_2 = .89 x 10 x 1.34 = 11.9 ml O_2/dl
      Patient (2) is slightly more hypoxemic

    b) (1) CaO_2 = .92 x 15 x 1.34 = 18.5 ml O_2/dl
       (2) CaO_2 = .92 x 15 x 1.34 = 18.5 ml O_2/dl
      The patients have equal amounts of hemoglobin-bound
      oxygen content

    c) (1) CaO_2 = .90 x 12 x 1.34 = 14.5 ml O_2/dl
       (2) CaO_2 = .80 x 12 x 1.34 = 12.9 ml O_2/dl
      Patient (2) is more hypoxemic

    d) (1) CaO_2 = .98 x 12 x 1.34 = 15.8 ml O_2/dl
       (2) CaO_2 = .90 x 12 x 1.34 = 14.5 ml O_2/dl
      Patient (2) is more hypoxemic

5-4.   For this question you have to find the SaO_2 for some of
       the PaO_2 values from a standard oxygen dissociation
       curve, then subtract the CO level to arrive at the true
       SaO_2.

    a)   (1) CaO_2 = .78 x 15 x 1.34 = 15.7 ml O_2/dl
          (2) CaO_2 = .98 x 12 x 1.34 = 15.8 ml O_2/dl
         The oxygen contents are almost identical; however
         patient (1), with 20% CO, is more *hypoxic* because
         of the left-shift of the O_2-dissociation curve.

    b)   (1) CaO_2 = .94 x 15 x 1.34 = 18.9 ml O_2/dl
          (2) CaO_2 = .85 x 15 x 1.34 = 17.1 ml O_2/dl
         Patient (2) is more hypoxemic

(continued)

Answers to numbered questions (continued)

5-4. (continued)

    c)   (1) CaO_2 = .90 x 5 x .1.34 = 6.0 ml O_2/dl
           (2) CaO_2 = .78 x 15 x 1.34 = 15.7 ml O_2/dl
           Patient (1) is more hypoxemic, because of severe anemia.

    d)   (1) CaO_2 = .87 x 10 x .1.34 = 11.7 ml O_2/dl
           (2) CaO_2 = .83 x 15 x 1.34 = 16.7 ml O_2/dl
           Patient (1) is more hypoxemic.

5-5.   Virtually any amount of CO could be in this patient's blood (although the fact that he came to the ED without assistance suggests the level is < 40%). Pulse oximetry "reads" carboxyhemoglobin and oxyhemoglobin together and reports the two values as "SaO_2."

5-6.   Answers for this problem require use of both the alveolar gas and oxygen content equations. Because of the high FIO_2 values, the factor 1.2 is dropped from the alveolar gas equation. Also, we can assume that SaO_2 = 100% minus the %COHb. Unlike the other problems presented so far, we cannot ignore the contribution here of dissolved oxygen to the total oxygen content.

5-6.   a) FIO_2 at 80%, CO level down to 45%.

    PAO_2 = .8(713) - 30 mm Hg = 540 mm Hg
    PaO_2 = 540 - 50 = 490 mm Hg
    CaO_2 = (15 x .55 x 1.34) + (.003 x 540)
          = 11.1 + 1.6 = 12.7 ml O_2/dl

(continued)

Answers to numbered questions (continued)

5-6. (continued)

b) Intubated, on 100% oxygen, CO level down to 40%.

$PAO_2 = 1.0(760-47) - 30$ mm Hg $= 683$ mm Hg
$PaO_2 = 683 - 50 = 633$ mm Hg
$CaO_2 = (15$ x $.60$ x $1.34) + (.003$ x $633)$
$\quad\quad = 12.1 + 1.9 = 14.0$ ml O_2/dl

c) Placed in a hyperbaric chamber at two atmospheres pressure ($=1520$ mm Hg), on 100% O_2, CO level 40%.

$PAO_2 = 1.0(1520-47) - 30$ mm Hg $= 1443$ mm Hg
$PaO_2 = 1443 - 50 = 1393$ mm Hg
$CaO_2 = (15$ x $.60$ x $1.34) + (.003$ x $1393)$
$\quad\quad = 12.1 + 4.2 = 16.3$ ml O_2/dl

d) Placed in a hyperbaric chamber at three atmospheres pressure ($=2280$ mm Hg), on 50% O_2, CO level 30%.

$PAO_2 = 1.0(2280-47) - 30$ mm Hg $= 2203$ mm Hg
$PaO_2 = 2203 - 50 = 2153$ mm Hg
$CaO_2 = (15$ x $.70$ x $1.34) + (.003$ x $2153)$
$\quad\quad = 14.1 + 6.5 = 20.6$ ml O_2/dl

5-7. Assuming normal ventilation ($PaCO_2 = 40$ mm Hg) and a $P(A-a)O_2$ of 50 mm Hg, the following calculations show that one atmosphere of pressure places about 1.9 ml O_2/dl of dissolved oxygen in the blood when the subject is inhaling 100% oxygen.

$PAO_2 = 1.0(760-47) - 40$ mm Hg $= 673$ mm Hg
$PaO_2 = PAO_2 - 50$ mm Hg $= 623$ mm Hg
Dissolved O_2 content $= .003$ x $623 = 1.87$ ml O_2/dl

(continued)

Answers to numbered questions (continued)

5-7. (continued)

Each additional atmosphere delivers a slightly higher O_2 content because the $PaCO_2$ and water vapor pressure are subtracted only once. Thus the next atmosphere of oxygen pressure can contribute

.003 x 760 mm Hg = 2.3 ml O_2/dl.

Normal blood oxygen content is about 20 ml O_2/dl. Since each atmosphere at 100% FIO_2 delivers slightly over 2 ml O_2/dl to the blood, the correct answer is c, 9 atmospheres.

5-8.   When someone with a normal respiratory system breathes supplemental oxygen, the SpO_2 should be close to 100%. A fall in SpO_2 from 99% to 91% could be due to a precipitous fall in PaO_2 (e.g., from pulmonary aspiration), but such a condition would likely be accompanied by some respiratory distress. A more likely explanation is met-hemoglobinemia from topical airway anesthetic; such anesthetics are commonly used to facilitate insertion of the endoscope.

Once methemoglobinemia is suspected, the endoscopy procedure should be aborted and the patient examined for cyanosis, always present with modest methemoglobinemia. At the same time, the FIO_2 should be increased (by switching to a high flow oxygen face mask) and the patient watched carefully over the next 24 hours, both clinically and with arterial blood gas measurements. Specific treatment with a reducing agent (e.g., methylene blue) is not necessary unless the methemoglobin continues to increase and poses a threat to the patient. There is no minimal threshold that demands treatment, but it should be strongly considered if the methemoglobin exceeds 15%.

pH, $PaCO_2$, HCO_3^- and Acid-base Status

The Henderson-Hasselbalch equation and pH

Among the three physiologic processes assessed by blood gas data, acid-base is perhaps the most complicated. Oxygenation and ventilation problems can often be assessed by a single abnormal variable (e.g., PaO_2 or $PaCO_2$) and almost always arise from impairment in a single organ system (respiratory). By contrast, acid-base disorders require knowledge of two or more variables and they may arise from renal, pulmonary and/or gastrointestinal impairment, or from exogenous chemicals and poisons.

Carbon dioxide, a byproduct of metabolism, combines with water in the blood to form carbonic acid, H_2CO_3. Carbonic acid quickly dissociates into hydrogen ions and bicarbonate. These reactions are reversible, i.e., they may go either way.

$$CO_2 + H_2O \longleftrightarrow H_2CO_3 \longleftrightarrow H^+ + HCO_3^-$$

The concentration of hydrogen ion is related to the concentration of carbonic acid and bicarbonate. The Henderson-Hasselbalch (H-H) equation defines the hydrogen ion concentration in terms of pH as follows:

$$pH = pK + \log \frac{[HCO_3^-]}{[H_2CO_3]}$$

where pK is the negative logarithm of the dissociation constant for carbonic acid (6.1) and pH is the negative logarithm of hydrogen ion concentration ($[H^+]$) in nanomoles/liter (nM/L). Almost all $[H_2CO_3]$ in the blood is in the form of dissolved CO_2. To obtain a quantity for the denominator of the equation, $PaCO_2$ is multiplied by its solubility coefficient, 0.03 mEq/L/mm Hg. Thus we obtain the more familiar form of the H-H equation.

$$pH = pK + \log \frac{HCO_3^-}{0.03(PaCO_2)}$$

?
What is the normal ratio of HCO_3^- to $PaCO_2$ in the H-H equation?

Normal HCO_3^- is 24 mEq/L and normal $PaCO_2$ is 40 mm Hg; this $PaCO_2$ value times 0.03 = 1.2 mEq/L, so the normal ratio is 20 to one. The logarithm of 20 is 1.3 which, when added to the pK value of 6.1, gives the normal pH of 7.4.

Many people view pH, which is unitless, as an unnecessarily confusing term; not only does pH correlate *inversely* with $[H^+]$ but small numerical changes reflect large changes in $[H^+]$ (Table 6-1). There has been much debate in the literature on whether pH should be discarded in favor of $[H^+]$ as the clinical term for acidity. Whatever the merits of this argument, pH has remains in worldwide use and seems in no danger of yielding to $[H^+]$ in blood gas reports.

Table 6-1 shows the corresponding $[H^+]$ values for pH from 7.00 to 8.00 and the percent change between selected values. A pH of 7.40 = 40 nM/L $[H^+]$. An 0.1 unit *decrease* in pH from 7.40 to 7.30 represents a 25% *increase* in $[H^+]$ (Table 6-1). A similar percentage change in serum sodium would raise its value from a normal 140 to 175 mEq/L!

Table 6-1. pH and hydrogen ion concentration

Blood pH	$[H^+]$ (nM/L)	% Change from normal
Acidemia		
7.00	100	+ 150
7.10	80	+ 100
7.30	50	+ 25
Normal		
7.40	40	
Alkalemia		
7.52	30	- 25
7.70	20	- 50
8.00	10	- 75

Although practically everyone entering the clinical arena is taught the H-H equation at some point, outside blood gas labs the equation is seldom (if ever) used to calculate pH or any other variable. Why then such emphasis on this admittedly complicated equation? Clinical importance of the H-H equation relates to the following:

- The bicarbonate system is quantitatively the largest buffering system in the extracellular fluid; its buffer components (HCO_3^- and $PaCO_2$) instantly reflect any blood acid-base disturbance.

- The three variables in the H-H equation are easily measured (or two can be measured and the third calculated).

- The simple proportion in the equation

$$pH \sim \frac{HCO_3^-}{PaCO_2}$$

  can be used to describe the four primary acid-base disorders. The *change*, in degree and direction, of the two buffer components is the key to understanding acid-base disorders.

What is the pH of a blood sample with HCO_3^- 36 mEq/L and $PaCO_2$ 60 mm Hg?

?
a) 7.1   d) 7.5
b) 7.3   e) indeterminate without more data
c) 7.4

I wrote before that a calculator was not required when reading this book, so don't bother looking for one to calculate the logarithm in the H-H equation. In this question, both HCO_3^- and $PaCO_2$ are increased 50% above normal, but since the ratio of the two values is unchanged, the logarithm of the ratio and resulting pH are also unchanged. The correct answer is therefore 7.4.

What is the pH of a blood sample with HCO_3^- 16 mEq/L?

?
a) 7.1   d) 7.4
b) 7.3   e) indeterminate without more data
c) 7.4

The answer is indeterminate. You need to know two of the three H-H variables to obtain the third. In this example the blood could be acidemic or alkalemic.

What is the pH of a blood sample with HCO_3^- 24 mEq/L and $PaCO_2$ 80 mm Hg?

> ?
> a) 7.1   d) 7.5
> b) 7.3   e) 7.6
> c) 7.4

You could calculate pH from the H-H equation but it is unnecessary. A normal HCO_3^- with twice normal $PaCO_2$ will make the blood very acidic, far more than just pH 7.3, which is only 25% above baseline acidity (Table 6-1). The only reasonable answer among the choices given is pH 7.1.

Base excess vs. bicarbonate

One of the more confusing calculations coming from the blood gas lab is base excess, abbreviated BE. Most clinicians know BE is somehow related to bicarbonate concentration, $[HCO_3^-]$, but exactly how? BE is not really an essential value in interpreting arterial blood gases. However, BE is so frequently mentioned in either blood gas reports or textbooks, and is frequently a source of confusion, that space will be taken here to explain the term. This explanation should make you feel a little more comfortable in interpreting blood gas data that include BE.

Apart from bicarbonate, the blood contains other buffers, principally hemoglobin. When fixed acid is added to blood the total quantity of buffer base per liter, or [BB], *decreases* in proportion to the amount of added acid, just as bicarbonate decreases. Similarly, because bicarbonate is part of blood's total buffer base, [BB] also *increases* in states of metabolic alkalosis. In other words, any rise or fall of $[HCO_3^-]$ will be mirrored in a rise or fall of [BB].

In theory, [BB] should more accurately assess metabolic acid-base disturbances since it represents all the buffer base, not just [HCO_3^-]. Of course you have to know the patient's hemoglobin content ([Hb]) to determine [BB]. With normal [Hb] of 15 gm%, [BB] is about 48 mEq/L. When [Hb] is 8 gm%, [BB] is about 45 mEq/L.

Base excess is the difference between the patient's normal [BB] and his or her actual [BB]. Although originally based on *in vitro* titration of blood, and therefore a measurement, base excess as reported in blood gas labs today is actually a calculation. Hence,

$$BE = \text{normal [BB] - calculated [BB]}$$

Normally BE is zero +/- 2 mEq/L. If BE has a positive value (more than 2 mEq/L), the patient has an excess of the metabolic component and [HCO_3^-] should also be increased. If BE has a negative value (less than -2 mEq/L) the patient has a *base deficit* and [HCO_3^-] should also be decreased; sometimes this situation is referred to as "negative base excess," an admittedly confusing term.

Base excess is a complicated way of reporting that the metabolic component of the blood — of which bicarbonate is about half the total — is increased or decreased. Because BE takes into account all the buffer base, and not just bicarbonate, there is not a one-to-one or exact linear relationship between BE and bicarbonate.

The following data on one sample of arterial blood includes both bicarbonate and base excess. The BE of 15 mEq/L indicates a large increase in the metabolic component; this is also reflected in the calculated bicarbonate, which is 18 mEq/L above normal. Either value, *along with the pH and PaCO$_2$*, suggests two acid-base disorders: metabolic alkalosis and compensated respiratory acidosis.

pH	7.45
$PaCO_2$	62 mm Hg
PaO_2	73 mm Hg
HCO_3^-	42 mEq/L
SaO_2	93%
Hb	13.9 gm%
BE	15 mEq/L

There are four reasons why I don't emphasize base excess in teaching blood gas interpretation.

First, it has a confusing terminology, particularly when BE is negative and one hears the term "negative base excess."

Second, BE is a calculation, the equation for which may vary from lab to lab (some labs calculate BE for whole blood only, whereas other labs calculate BE for all the extracellular fluid). The formula is complicated and nothing any clinician needs to know, unlike the formulas for oxygen content or anion gap, for example. BE thus adds a layer of "mysticism" (where did this number come from?) and complexity to blood gas interpretation.

Third, in chronic respiratory disorders, where increases or decreases in bicarbonate may be appropriate, the abnormal BE may suggest a "metabolic problem" that requires attention. For example, the values pH 7.36, $PaCO_2$ 58 mm Hg, HCO_3^- 34 mEq/L may represent a patient's steady state of chronic respiratory acidosis; a BE of 12 mEq/L reported with these data suggests significant metabolic abnormality when in fact the metabolic response — renal retention of bicarbonate for compensation of respiratory acidosis — is desired and appropriate.

Fourth, by closely examining the calculated bicarbonate value, blood gases can be adequately interpreted without knowing the BE. Since not all labs report BE, but do calculate HCO_3^-, the clinician should become thoroughly familiar with interpreting acid-base status without BE. Facility in using the HCO_3^- should eliminate the need for calculating or worrying about base excess.

In summary, BE is a calculation based on the concept of how much the total base for the blood sample varies from the normal value; the result could be a positive or negative number (the latter called "negative base excess" or base deficit). BE does not take into account the appropriateness of the excess or deficit, and provides no more useful information than is provided by the calculated bicarbonate value. For these reasons BE will not be used throughout this book.

Clinical usefulness of the serum CO_2

In the blood gas lab, bicarbonate is calculated using the Henderson-Hasselbalch equation; $PaCO_2$ and pH are measured and the pK is assumed to be 6.1. By contrast, chemistry labs routinely *measure* bicarbonate in venous blood as a component of the serum electrolytes (along with Na^+, K^+ and Cl^-).

The measured venous bicarbonate includes the mEq/L contributed by dissolved CO_2, i.e., the $PaCO_2$, and is thus quantitatively different from what the blood gas lab calculates as HCO_3^-. When dissolved CO_2 exerts a partial pressure of 40 mm Hg in arterial blood, its *quantity* as a gas is

$$.03 \times 40 \text{ mm Hg} = 1.2 \text{ mEq/L.}$$

The clinical chemistry lab measures *both* the actual bicarbonate (numerator of H-H equation) and the quantity of dissolved CO_2 (denominator of the H-H equation), and reports the result as "CO_2" or "total CO_2" in mEq/L; this value obviously should not be confused with $PaCO_2$, which is the partial pressure of CO_2 as measured in the blood gas lab.

Although serum CO_2 should be within one or two mEq/L of the calculated arterial HCO_3^-, the difference is often much greater and can occur *in both directions*. Table 6-2 lists some reasons why the two values often differ by more than one or two mEq/L, and why either value may be higher or lower than the other.

Table 6-2. Reasons why calculated HCO_3^- may differ from measured CO_2

1. Venous HCO_3^- normally runs slightly higher than arterial HCO_3^-.
2. Arterial HCO_3^- is calculated using a pK value of 6.1; venous value is measured as part of the total CO_2 (which includes contribution of $PaCO_2$).
3. The true pK may vary from the assumed value of 6.1 in critically ill patients (Hood 1982).
4. Arterial and venous blood are usually drawn at different times and the patient's acid-base state may have changed in interim.
5. Venous blood may sit in a test tube open to air before it is measured, thereby losing some CO_2 to diffusion.
6. The blood-drawing technique may alter venous CO_2, e.g., tourniquet placement may create a transient lactic acidosis, lowering the venous HCO_3^-.
7. If pH and/or $PaCO_2$ are inaccurately measured, the calculated HCO_3^- will be inaccurate as well.

6-1. A 54-year-old man is hospitalized with congestive heart failure. The blood gas lab reports arterial pH 7.52, $PaCO_2$ 44 mm Hg, HCO_3^- 34 mEq/L. A venous CO_2 measured at the same time is 24 mEq/L. What is his acid-base status?

Although two of the three H-H variables are needed to determine the third, an isolated value can be clinically useful. If any one of the three H-H variables is truly abnormal, the patient must have an acid-base disturbance of some type. Therefore, assuming no lab or transcription error, *a high or low calculated HCO₃⁻ or measured CO₂ indicates an acid-base disorder.* Since electrolytes are measured far more often than blood gases, serum CO_2 is often the first clue to an underlying acid-base disorder. Overlooking an abnormal CO_2 value can lead to serious clinical error.

Refer to the case presented in Chapter 3, page 35. At the time the sedative was ordered there were two venous CO_2 measurements in that patient's chart, both elevated at 34 mEq/L. From the limited information provided, what do you think explains that patient's elevated CO_2 value?

?
a) metabolic alkalosis
b) respiratory acidosis with renal compensation
c) normal value for an elderly patient
d) laboratory error

Abnormality of a single H-H variable can arise from *two or more* acid-base disorders. For example, an elevated HCO_3^- or serum CO_2 can occur from metabolic alkalosis, or respiratory acidosis, or both. Lab error, always a possibility, is less likely when two separate measurements are in close agreement. No arterial blood gas was obtained while the patient was in the regular medical ward, but it was probably assumed that her elevated CO_2 reflected mild metabolic alkalosis (from prior diuretic therapy). The patient had a long history of smoking but respiratory acidosis was not considered. In fact, her elevated CO_2 reflected a state of chronic respiratory acidosis with renal compensation.

When she arrived in the ICU her pH was 7.07, $PaCO_2$ 83 mm Hg and HCO_3^- 23 mEq/L, values that reflected a worsening of the previously unrecognized respiratory acidosis *plus* a new metabolic acidosis (lactic acidosis from poor organ perfusion). Her anxiety just before the ICU transfer was related to worsening respiratory acidosis and dyspnea.

The anion gap

Venous CO_2 is also useful as part of the anion gap calculation:

$$AG = Na^+ - (Cl^- + CO_2)$$

The normal AG calculated in this manner is 12 +/- 4 mEq/L. The anion gap exists simply because not all electrolytes are routinely measured; the quantity of routinely measured cations (Na^+ and K^+) is 8 to 16 mEq/L greater than that of routinely measured anions (Cl^- and CO_2). (If AG is calculated using K^+ the normal gap is 16 +/- 4 mEq/L.)

Unmeasured anions include phosphates, sulfates and anionic proteins. If *all* the cations and anions in the blood were measured, the two groups would be equal in concentration and there would be no anion gap.

An *elevated* AG occurs when an excess quantity of unmeasured anion enters the blood. Examples include the anions of lactic acid, ketoacids, aspirin, and metabolites of some drugs like paraldehyde. Because all excess anions in the blood are buffered by bicarbonate, an elevated AG indicates a state of metabolic acidosis (Gabow 1980, Gabow 1985, Oster 1988). This is true even if the actual measured serum CO_2 is normal or above normal.

> ?
> A 42-year-old man is admitted to the hospital with dehydration and hypotension. Electrolytes show Na^+ 165 mEq/L, K^+ 4.0 mEq/L, CO_2 32 mEq/L, Cl^- 112 mEq/L. No arterial blood gas is obtained. Does this patient have metabolic acidosis?

This patient's anion gap is 165 - (32 + 112) = 21 mEq/L. Despite the fact that his CO_2 is elevated (reflecting a metabolic alkalosis from dehydration), there is *also* a slight metabolic acidosis, from hypotension and poor tissue perfusion.

As we have seen, any truly abnormal HCO_3^- or CO_2 value indicates some type of acid-base disorder. An increase in the AG can point to a metabolic acidosis irrespective of the actual value of the (calculated) HCO_3^- or (measured) CO_2.

> 6-2. A patient with a $PaCO_2$ of 50 mm Hg and an anion gap of 20 mEq/L has the following electrolyte values: Na^+ 145 mEq/L, Cl^- 104 mEq/L. From this information, how could you calculate the pH?

Relationships among the H-H variables

The simple relationship of pH to the ratio of HCO_3^- over $PaCO_2$ can be used to describe the four primary acid-base disorders and their compensatory changes (Figure 6-1). In describing any acid-base disorder, distinction should be made between changes in the blood and changes in the patient; the former go by the terms *acidemia* and *alkalemia*, the latter by the terms *acidosis* and *alkalosis* (Winters 1965). The reason for this important distinction will become clearer when we discuss mixed acid-base disorders. Some definitions are given below.

Acidemia: present when blood pH < 7.35

Acidosis: a primary physiologic process that, occurring alone, tends to cause acidemia. Examples: metabolic acidosis from low-perfusion lactic acidosis; respiratory acidosis from acute hypoventilation. If the patient also has an alkalosis at the same time, the resulting blood pH may be low, normal or high.

Alkalemia: present when blood pH > 7.45

Alkalosis: a primary physiologic process that, occurring alone, tends to cause alkalemia. Examples: metabolic alkalosis from excessive diuretic therapy; respiratory alkalosis from acute hyperventilation. If the patient also has an acidosis at the same time, the resulting blood pH may be high, normal or low.

Figure 6-1. The four primary acid-base disorders and their compensatory changes. The primary event leads to a large change in pH (larger arrows). Compensation (changes in HCO_3^- and $PaCO_2$ represented by smaller arrows) attempts to normalize the ratio of $HCO_3^-/PaCO_2$ and bring the pH back toward normal (smaller arrows next to pH). Each primary disorder may be caused by a variety of specific clinical conditions (see Table 6-3).

PRIMARY EVENT   COMPENSATORY EVENT

Metabolic acidosis

$$\downarrow pH \cong \frac{\downarrow HCO_3^-}{PaCO_2} \qquad \downarrow pH \cong \frac{\downarrow HCO_3^-}{\downarrow PaCO_2}$$

Metabolic alkalosis

$$\uparrow pH \cong \frac{\uparrow HCO_3^-}{PaCO_2} \qquad \uparrow pH \cong \frac{\uparrow HCO_3^-}{\uparrow PaCO_2}$$

Respiratory acidosis

$$\downarrow pH \cong \frac{HCO_3^-}{\uparrow PaCO_2} \qquad \downarrow pH \cong \frac{\uparrow HCO_3^-}{\uparrow PaCO_2}$$

Respiratory alkalosis

$$\uparrow pH \cong \frac{HCO_3^-}{\downarrow PaCO_2} \qquad \uparrow pH \cong \frac{\downarrow HCO_3^-}{\downarrow PaCO_2}$$

Primary acid-base disorder: One of the four acid-base disturbances manifested by an initial change in either HCO_3^- or $PaCO_2$ (Figure 6-1). If HCO_3^- is first to change, the disorder is either a metabolic acidosis (reduced HCO_3^-; acidemia) or metabolic alkalosis (elevated HCO_3^-; alkalemia). If the $PaCO_2$ is first to change, the problem is either respiratory alkalosis (reduced $PaCO_2$; alkalemia) or respiratory acidosis (elevated $PaCO_2$; acidemia).

Compensation: The change in HCO_3^- or $PaCO_2$ that occurs as a result of the primary event. Compensatory changes are not classified by the terms acidosis or alkalosis. For example, a patient who hyperventilates (lowers $PaCO_2$) solely as compensation for metabolic acidosis does *not* have a respiratory alkalosis. Since the hyperventilation occurs solely as compensation for metabolic acidosis there is no respiratory alkalosis, the latter being a primary disorder that, alone, would lead to alkalemia. In uncomplicated metabolic acidosis the patient will never develop alkalemia.

The four primary acid-base disorders and their clinical causes

The diagnosis of any primary acid-base disorder is analogous to diagnoses like "anemia" or "fever"; a specific cause must be sought in order to provide proper treatment. Each primary acid-base disorder (Figure 6-1) arises from one or more specific clinical conditions, although the specific clinical cause may not be readily apparent. Table 6-3 lists the most common clinical conditions that lead to acid-base disturbances.

Respiratory alkalosis and respiratory acidosis

Any discussion of primary acid base disorders should begin with respiratory alkalosis and acidosis. Together, these two disorders characterize the body's "titration" of carbon dioxide. Table 6-4 shows the changes in HCO_3^- and pH as $PaCO_2$ rises from 15 to 90 mm Hg. These data, generated experimentally on human subjects in two separate studies (Brackett 1965, Arbus 1969), are also graphed as the bands for acute respiratory alkalosis and acidosis shown on the acid-base map, Figure 6-2.

For the low $PaCO_2$ band (acute respiratory alkalosis), subjects were hyperventilated during anesthesia for elective surgery; their arterial blood gases were measured within 10 minutes. For the high $PaCO_2$ band (acute respiratory acidosis) healthy volunteers were placed in an environmental chamber and given 5% CO_2 to inhale; their blood gases were also measured within 10 minutes.

Table 6-3. Clinical causes of the four primary acid-base disorders

Metabolic acidosis
with increased anion gap
  lactic acidosis
  ketoacidosis
  poisoning, e.g., paraldehyde, methanol, aspirin
with normal anion gap
  diarrhea
  renal tubular acidosis
  excess NH$_4$Cl administration
  drainage from a ureterosigmoidostomy
  acetazolamide administration

Metabolic alkalosis
  diuretics
  corticosteroids
  nasogastric suctioning
  vomiting of gastric contents
  severe dehydration

Respiratory acidosis (= respiratory failure)
  central nervous system depression, e.g., drug overdose, anesthesia
  chest bellows weakness or dysfunction, e.g., myasthenia gravis, polio,
    massive obesity, diaphragm paralysis, flail chest, administration of
    paralyzing agents
  disease of lungs and/or upper airway, e.g., severe asthma attack, chronic
    obstructive pulmonary disease, severe pneumonia, severe pulmonary
    edema, upper airway obstruction

Respiratory alkalosis
  voluntary hyperventilation
  hypoxemia (includes altitude)
  liver failure
  anxiety
  sepsis
  any acute pulmonary problem, e.g., acute pulmonary embolism,
    pneumonia, mild asthma attack, mild pulmonary edema

Table. 6-4. Changes in pH and HCO_3^- with acute changes in $PaCO_2$ (Data from Brackett, Arbus 1965).

Data for each $PaCO_2$ value represent the 95% confidence limits for pH and bicarbonate when $PaCO_2$ changes acutely (before any renal compensation takes place); 95% of all subjects with acute hyperventilation or hypoventilation to the degree shown, and no other acid-base disorder(s), should have blood gas values within these ranges. Note that bicarbonate decreases with acute hyperventilation and increases with acute hypoventilation. These data are graphed in Figure 6-2 as the bands for acute respiratory alkalosis and acute respiratory acidosis.

$PaCO_2$ (mm Hg)	pH	HCO_3^- (mEq/L)
15	7.61 - 7.74	15.3 - 20.5
20	7.55 - 7.66	17.7 - 22.8
30	7.45 - 7.53	21.0 - 25.6
40	7.38 - 7.45	22.8 - 26.8
50	7.31 - 7.36	24.1 - 27.5
60	7.24 - 7.29	25.1 - 27.9
70	7.19 - 7.23	25.7 - 28.5
80	7.14 - 7.18	26.2 - 28.9
90	7.13 - 7.09	26.5 - 29.2

Figure 6-2 (next page). Acid-base map showing confidence bands for the four primary acid-base disorders, plus the bands for chronic respiratory acidosis and chronic respiratory alkalosis. Human titration curve for carbon dioxide is a continuous band made by joining the bands for acute respiratory alkalosis (in this figure, $PaCO_2$ from 10 to 40 mm Hg) and acidosis ($PaCO_2$ from 40 to 100 mm Hg); see also Table 6-2. (From Goldberg M, Green SB, Moss ML, et al: JAMA 223: 269-275, 1973, copyright 1973, American Medical Association.)

Figure 6-2 (legend page 116).

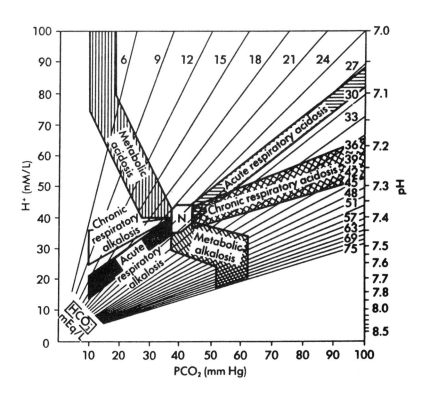

The CO_2 titration band is especially useful in the presence of mixed acid-base disorders. Respiratory disorders with blood gas values falling outside the band indicate that a) the problem is not acute or b) the problem may be mixed.

6-3. A patient's arterial blood gas shows a pH of 7.14, $PaCO_2$ of 70 mm Hg, and HCO_3^- of 23 mEq/L. How would you describe the likely acid-base disorder(s)?

Metabolic acidosis

Metabolic acidosis is conveniently divided into increased and normal anion gap acidosis (Table 6-3). Increased anion gap acidosis arises from excess acid added to the blood that has an unmeasured anion, e.g., lactic acidosis (lactate anion). Normal AG acidosis arises from: acid added to the blood where the excess anion is chloride, which is routinely measured (e.g., NH_4Cl administration); or loss of bicarbonate from the blood (e.g., profuse diarrhea, renal tubular acidosis) that is replaced by chloride.

The expected human compensation (95% confidence band) for metabolic acidosis is shown in Figure 6-2. This band was generated from patients with uncomplicated metabolic acidosis (e.g., diabetic ketoacidosis) who had been in this state for at least 24 hours (Asch 1969, Pierce 1970). Any patient with metabolic acidosis whose blood gas values fall outside this band likely has either 1) very early metabolic acidosis (before full compensation has taken place) or 2) a mixed acid-base disorder.

Metabolic alkalosis

Metabolic alkalosis can occur from excess bicarbonate added to the blood, or from loss of HCl. Excess bicarbonate can occur from exogenous administration or from excess renal reabsorption (as seen with diuretic therapy). Loss of HCl is commonly seen with nasogastric suctioning and vomiting.

Unlike the other primary acid-base disorders, there is no narrow confidence band for metabolic alkalosis; the one shown in Figure 6-2 encompasses both normal and high $PaCO_2$ values. The degree of change in $PaCO_2$ from pure metabolic alkalosis is wide ranging. Recent studies have actually described two broad compensation bands for this disorder, depending on the severity of bicarbonate elevation (Javaheri 1982, Javaheri 1987).

Does the patient have a mixed acid-base disorder?

There is perhaps no more confusing topic related to blood gases than mixed acid-base disorders. Acid-base maps such as the one in Figure 6-2 are often brought out to help unravel mixed disorders. Although these maps and similar visual aids are helpful (if readily available and used properly, which is not always the case), the clinical history plus basic blood gas and electrolyte data often suffice to "figure out" most mixed disorders.

Specific changes in pH, $PaCO_2$ and HCO_3^- in single acid-base disorders, except perhaps for metabolic alkalosis, occur in a fairly predictable fashion, making it possible to spot the presence of mixed disorders. I have found the following 32 "tips" especially helpful in clinical practice.

TIP 1. Single acid-base disorders do not lead to normal blood pH. Although pH can end up in the normal range (7.35 - 7.45) with single disorders of a mild degree, a truly normal pH with distinctly abnormal HCO_3^- and $PaCO_2$ invariably suggests two or more primary disorders. Example: pH 7.40, $PaCO_2$ 20 mm Hg, HCO_3^- 12 mEq/L. These blood gas data were from a patient with sepsis, who had *both* acute respiratory alkalosis and metabolic acidosis. Although pH is normal it resulted from two acute and unstable acid-base disorders.

TIP 2. The bicarbonate level changes with acute changes in $PaCO_2$ (Table 6-4). This observation is perhaps the most useful in diagnosing the presence of a mixed acid-base disorder. Acute CO_2 retention (i.e., acute hypoventilation) drives the hydration reaction (shown on page 101) to the right and as a result, HCO_3^- increases slightly. Acute CO_2 excretion (i.e., acute hyperventilation) drives the hydration equation to the left and HCO_3^- decreases slightly. As already pointed out, these changes in HCO_3^- are instantaneous and have *nothing* to do with the kidneys or renal compensation. Thus:

a)   a normal or slightly low HCO_3^- in the presence of hypercapnia indicates a concomitant metabolic acidosis, e.g., pH 7.27, $PaCO_2$ 50 mm Hg, HCO_3^- 22 mEq/L;

b)   a normal or slightly elevated HCO_3^- in the presence of hypocapnia indicates a concomitant metabolic alkalosis, e.g., pH 7.56, $PaCO_2$ 30 mm Hg, HCO_3^- 26 mEq/L.

TIP 3.   Acute respiratory disorders up to a point can be expressed by simplified rules that predict the pH and HCO_3^- for a given change in $PaCO_2$. If the pH or HCO_3^- is higher or lower than expected, the patient probably has an additional metabolic acid-base disorder. The following rules are an approximation of the data provided in Table 6-4.

a)   in acute respiratory acidosis up to $PaCO_2$ 70 mm Hg:
for every 10 mm Hg ↑ in $PaCO_2$ . . .
pH ↓ by 0.07 units and HCO_3^- ↑ by one mEq/L.

b)   in acute respiratory alkalosis down to $PaCO_2$ 20 mm Hg:
for every 10 mm Hg ↓ in $PaCO_2$ . . .
pH ↑ by 0.08 units and HCO_3^- ↓ by 2 mEq/L.

TIP 4. In fully compensated metabolic acidosis, the numerical value of $PaCO_2$ should be the same (or close to) the last two digits of arterial pH (Narins 1980).

Given the following blood gas values, what is (are) the likely acid-base disorder(s)?

?
a) pH 7.28, $PaCO_2$ 50 mm Hg, HCO_3^- 23 mEq/L

b) pH 7.50, $PaCO_2$ 33 mm Hg, HCO_3^- 25 mEq/L

c) pH 7.25, $PaCO_2$ 30 mm Hg, HCO_3^- 14 mEq/L

In the first example the bicarbonate is lower than expected for acute CO_2 retention; the patient has respiratory acidosis *and* an accompanying metabolic acidosis. In the second example bicarbonate is higher than expected for acute hyperventilation; the patient has respiratory alkalosis *and* an accompanying metabolic alkalosis. In the third example $PaCO_2$ is higher than expected for fully compensated metabolic acidosis; this suggests a concomitant respiratory disorder or very early metabolic acidosis.

Always keep in mind that *any* isolated set of blood gas values can be explained by two or more co-existing acid-base disorders. Thus, even when blood gases fall into one of the 95% confidence bands, the patient *may* have a mixed disorder. Often, the only way to know for sure is by detailed analysis of all the clinical and laboratory information and close patient followup.

?

Explain the acid-base status of a 35-year-old man admitted to hospital with the following blood gas and electrolyte values: pH 7.52, $PaCO_2$ 30 mm Hg, PaO_2 62 mm Hg; Na^+ 142 mEq/L, Cl^- 98 mEq/L, K^+ 2.9 mEq/L; CO_2 21 mEq/L. The patient has fever and pneumonia.

The pH and $PaCO_2$ fit into the band of acute respiratory alkalosis. The patient has moderate hypoxemia and the blood gas data alone could be explained by acute hyperventilation due to his pneumonia. But the anion gap is elevated at 23 mEq/L, suggesting a concomitant metabolic acidosis. In fact the patient manifests *three separate* acid-base disorders: respiratory alkalosis (from pneumonia); metabolic acidosis (from renal disease); and hypokalemic metabolic alkalosis (from excessive diuretic therapy). The result? Blood gas values that are indistinguishable from those of uncomplicated acute respiratory alkalosis.

6-4. A 45-year-old man comes to hospital complaining of dyspnea that began a few days earlier. Arterial blood gas reveals pH 7.35, $PaCO_2$ 60 mm Hg, PaO_2 57 mm Hg, HCO_3^- 31 mEq/L. How would you characterize his acid-base status?

6-5. A 53-year-old man initially presents to the emergency department with the following blood gas values (FIO$_2$ .21): pH 7.51, PaCO$_2$ 50 mm Hg, PaO$_2$ 40 mm Hg, HCO$_3^-$ 39 mEq/L. His acid-base disorder is best characterized as:

a) metabolic alkalosis
b) metabolic alkalosis plus respiratory acidosis
c) respiratory acidosis with metabolic compensation
d) indeterminate without more information

He is found to have congestive heart failure and is treated with supplemental oxygen and diuretics. Three days later he is clinically improved, with pH 7.38, PaCO$_2$ 60 mm Hg, HCO$_3^-$ 34 mEq/L, and PaO$_2$ 73 mm Hg (on FIO$_2$ 24%). How would you characterize his acid-base status at this point?

6-6. The following laboratory values are found in a 65-year-old patient.

Arterial blood gas		Electrolytes, blood urea nitrogen (BUN), Glucose	
pH	7.51	Na$^+$	155 mEq/L
PaCO$_2$	50 mm Hg	K$^+$	5.5 mEq/L
HCO$_3^-$	39 mEq/L	Cl$^-$	90 mEq/L
		CO$_2$	40 mEq/L
		BUN	121 mgm%
		Glucose	77 mgm%

Which of the following most closely describes this patient's acid-base status?

a) severe metabolic acidosis
b) severe respiratory acidosis
c) respiratory acidosis plus metabolic alkalosis
d) metabolic alkalosis plus metabolic acidosis
e) respiratory acidosis plus respiratory alkalosis

6-7. A 52-year-old woman has been artificially ventilated for two days following a drug overdose. Her arterial blood gas values, stable for the past 12 hours, show pH 7.45, $PaCO_2$ 25 mm Hg. Serum electrolytes were Na^+ 142 mEq/L, CO_2 18 mEq/L, Cl^- 100 mEq/L, K^+ 4 mEq/L. How would you assess her acid-base status?

6-8. An 18-year-old girl is admitted to the ICU for an acute asthma attack, unabated to treatment received in the emergency department. ABG values (on room air) show: pH 7.45, $PaCO_2$ 25 mm Hg, HCO_3^- 17 mEq/L, PaO_2 55 mm Hg, SaO_2 87%. Her peak expiratory flow rate is 95 L/min (25% of predicted value). She continues to receive asthma medication. Two hours later she becomes more tired and her peak flow is now less than 60 L/minute. Blood gas values (on 40% oxygen) now show: pH 7.20, $PaCO_2$ 52 mm Hg, HCO_3^- 20 mEq/L, PaO_2 65 mm Hg. At this point intubation and artificial ventilation are considered. What is her acid-base status?

6-9. A 72-year-old man is admitted in shock, with 70 mm systolic blood pressure. He has a history of chronic obstructive pulmonary disease and takes medication for a heart condition. Initial arterial blood gas results (FIO_2 .40): $PaCO_2$ 70 mm Hg, pH 7.1, HCO_3^- 21 mEq/L, PaO_2 35 mm Hg, SaO_2 58 mm Hg. He is intubated and a subsequent blood gas analysis (on the same FIO_2) shows pH 7.30, $PaCO_2$ 40 mm Hg, PaO_2 87 mm Hg, HCO_3^- 19 mEq/L. His anion gap is elevated at 22 mEq/L. What is his acid-base status?

6-10. In review, state whether each of the following six statements is true or false.

a) Metabolic acidosis is always present when the measured CO_2 changes acutely from 24 to 21 mEq/L.

b) In acute respiratory acidosis, bicarbonate initially rises because of the reaction of CO_2 with water and the resultant formation of H_2CO_3.

c) If pH and $PaCO_2$ are both above normal, the calculated bicarbonate must also be above normal.

d) A serum CO_2 value above normal, if accurately measured, always indicates an acid-base disorder.

e) The compensation for chronic elevation of $PaCO_2$ is renal excretion of bicarbonate.

f) A normal pH with abnormal HCO_3^- or $PaCO_2$ suggests the presence of two or more acid-base disorders.

Summary — Clinical approach to acid-base diagnosis

Each primary acid-base disorder should be viewed as a physiologic process caused by a specific clinical problem or disease, not simply as changes in blood gas values. This view allows for unraveling complex or mixed acid-base disorders. Steps to proper acid-base diagnosis and management include:

- determine that the patient has an acid-base disorder from arterial blood gas and/or serum electrolyte measurements.

- use a full clinical assessment (history, physical examination, other laboratory data) to explain the disorder in terms of physiologic processes and underlying clinical condition(s).

- aim toward correcting the pH, particularly if it is outside the range of 7.30-7.52 ($[H^+] = 50\text{-}30$ nMole/L). The danger to the patient is not the absolute value of HCO_3^- or $PaCO_2$, but the abnormal pH.

- treat the underlying clinical condition.

Answers to numbered questions

6-1. There is a 10 mEq/L discrepancy between the calculated arterial HCO_3^- and measured serum CO_2. If pH and $PaCO_2$ are correct, so is the calculated HCO_3^-. Of course, either the pH or $PaCO_2$ may be measured incorrectly and then the HCO_3^- will also be incorrect. These blood gas values suggest a state of metabolic alkalosis (elevated HCO_3^-); the measured venous CO_2 is normal and does not agree with the blood gas HCO_3^-. Possible reasons for this large difference are listed in Table 6-2.

6-2. Assume the venous bicarbonate and the arterial bicarbonate are equal. Calculate the venous CO_2:

Anion gap $= Na^+ - (Cl^- + CO_2) = 20$ mEq/L

Since 20 mEq/L $= 145 - (104 + CO_2)$,

$CO_2 = 21$ mEq/L

You can now calculate pH from the H-H equation.

$$pH = 6.1 + \log \frac{21}{.03(50)} = 7.25$$

6-3. Acute elevation of $PaCO_2$ leads to reduced pH, i.e., an acute respiratory acidosis. However, is the problem *only* acute respiratory acidosis or is there some additional process? For every 10 mm Hg rise in $PaCO_2$ (before any renal compensation), pH falls about 0.07 units. Because this patient's pH is down 0.26, or 0.05 more than expected for a 30 mm Hg increase in $PaCO_2$, there must be an additional, metabolic problem.

(continued)

Answers to numbered questions (continued)

6.3. (continued)

Also note that the calculated HCO_3^- is low normal. With acute CO_2 retention, the HCO_3^- should be *elevated* 2 to 3 mEq/L; a low-normal HCO_3^- is another piece of evidence to suggest an additional, metabolic disorder. Decreased vascular perfusion leading to mild lactic acidosis would explain the metabolic component.

6-4. $PaCO_2$ and HCO_3^- are elevated, so the problem is more than uncomplicated acute respiratory acidosis. Since the patient has been dyspneic for several days it is fair to assume a chronic acid-base disorder. Most likely this patient has a chronic or partially compensated respiratory acidosis. Without electrolyte data, you cannot rule out an accompanying metabolic disorder.

6-5. Here the answer must be d, "indeterminate without more information." If an acid-base disorder is found (from blood gas, electrolyte data), the next logical step is to determine the clinical causes(s). Elevated $PaCO_2$, pH and HCO_3^- certainly suggest a metabolic alkalosis, but there are other possibilities. Isolated blood gas values should be viewed as a single point on a plot that can be arrived at from various pathways, and not as diagnostic of any particular acid-base disorder. Making a diagnosis of "metabolic alkalosis" solely on the basis of blood gas values has two potential pitfalls.

PITFALL 1. It suggests a final diagnosis, which is not the case. There are several causes of metabolic alkalosis and the *clinical reason* has to be found and corrected. Acidosis and alkalosis, with their adjectives metabolic and respiratory, are analogous to "anemia"

(continued)

Answers to numbered questions (continued)

6-5. (continued)

or "fever." Acidosis and alkalosis should always be viewed as mani-festations of underlying clinical problems and never as clinical diagnoses in themselves.

PITFALL 2. The patient may *not* have metabolic alkalosis or may have metabolic alkalosis *plus* another serious acid-base disorder. In fact, this patient's initial blood gas values represent several clinical possibilities — uncomplicated metabolic alkalosis, chronic respiratory acidosis followed by acute hyperventilation (acute respiratory alkalosis), and respiratory acidosis complicated by metabolic alkalosis. For example, suppose the patient's pulmonary function tests and blood gas values were normal one week earlier and in the interval he had taken diuretics; a *primary metabolic alkalosis* would then be the most likely diagnosis. On the other hand, he could be a patient with chronic CO_2 retention, e.g., $PaCO_2$ 60 mm Hg and pH 7.41; he then develops pneumonia and hyperventilates, lowering $PaCO_2$ from 60 to 50 mm Hg and raising pH above normal. This last situation would reflect a state of chronic respiratory acidosis plus an acute increase in ventilation (respiratory alkalosis), not a primary metabolic alkalosis. Thus the patient could have an isolated metabolic problem, an isolated resp-iratory problem, or a combination. Only by a detailed clinical and laboratory history, including previous blood gas data if available, can the actual cause be determined.

(continued)

Answers to numbered questions (continued)

6-5. (continued)

> After treatment for congestive heart failure, his baseline arterial blood gas values reflect a state of chronic respiratory acidosis. In retrospect, his blood gas values on admission were the result of acute hyperventilation on top of chronic respiratory acidosis.

6-6. The answer is d: metabolic alkalosis plus metabolic acidosis.   A patient can have both vomiting (causing metabolic alkalosis) as well as uremia (causing metabolic acidosis) at the same time.   This patient has renal failure (BUN 121 mgm%) with the diagnosis of metabolic acidosis confirmed by the elevated anion gap (25 mEq/L), even though the blood was alkalemic (pH 7.51).

From the information provided one cannot rule out a primary respiratory acidosis as an additional problem. (After this patient recovered he showed no evidence of underlying lung disease. Sometimes it requires days or weeks of followup to fully characterize acid base disorders.)

6-7. This patient's blood gas values suggest a state of chronic respiratory alkalosis: very low $PaCO_2$, slightly elevated pH.   However this assessment does not indicate a specific diagnosis but only suggests possibilities. Accurate diagnosis must be made in conjunction with the clinical picture plus other laboratory studies. Could this patient have a mixed problem — respiratory alkalosis plus metabolic acidosis? Her anion gap is

$$Na^+ - (Cl^- + CO_2) = 142 - 118 = 24 \text{ mEq/L.}$$

(continued)

Answers to numbered questions (continued)

6-7. (continued)

The anion gap is elevated and indicates a metabolic acidosis. However, the acid-base disorder is not *just* metabolic acidosis since the blood is alkalemic. There is good evidence she has *both* metabolic acidosis *and* respiratory alkalosis, the latter disorder from excessive artificial ventilation. The cause of metabolic acidosis must be looked for since it is not apparent from the information provided. Since the anion gap is elevated, the possibilities include lactic acidosis from hypoperfusion and drug-induced metabolic acidosis.

6-8. The patient initially had chronic respiratory alkalosis, resulting from several days of hyperventilation, during which time her kidneys had a chance to excrete bicarbonate and return the pH toward normal. Now her asthmatic condition has worsened; she has acutely hypoventilated. The second set of blood gas values reflects acute respiratory acidosis *in addition to* chronic respiratory alkalosis. Although her bicarbonate is low, there is no primary metabolic process and treatment must be aimed at her respiratory disorders.

6-9. This patient has more than respiratory acidosis because the initial calculated bicarbonate is low (21 mEq/L). There is a concomitant metabolic acidosis, confirmed by an elevated anion gap. He has two causes of metabolic acidosis: shock and severe hypoxemia. After intubation he is ventilated down to a "normal" $PaCO_2$ of 40 mm Hg, yet remains acidemic because his metabolic process (lactic acidosis) has not been corrected. The last set of blood gas values still shows metabolic acidosis and inadequate respiratory compensation.

Answers to numbered questions (continued)

6-10.   a) false
               b) true
               c) true
               d) true
               e) false
               f) true

CHAPTER 7.

Putting It All Together: Cases

You are now ready to interpret arterial blood gases in almost any clinical situation.   In this chapter are five actual cases managed with the aid of arterial blood gas data.   Each case is accompanied by multiple choice questions.   For each question select the *one best answer* (answers with explanations are at end of the chapter).   Remember to use *all available information* in answering each question.   For each case, I recommend you answer all the questions first, then check the answers.

__MR. A: A CASE OF ACUTE RESPIRATORY DISTRESS__. Mr. A is a 25-year-old man who comes to the emergency room complaining of increasing shortness of breath. He has had upper respiratory symptoms, mainly cough, fever and progressive dyspnea, for three days. On examination he appears cyanotic and in respiratory distress; inspiratory rales are heard over the left lung bases and his respiratory rate is 40/min.   Chest x-ray confirms a left lower lobe pneumonia. His temperature is 102°F, white blood cell count 17,000/mm^3. Serum electrolytes are normal except for a CO_2 of 20 mEq/L.   Arterial blood gas results, obtained with the patient breathing room air, show

pH	7.55
$PaCO_2$	25 mm Hg
PaO_2	38 mm Hg
SaO_2	78%
HCO_3^-	21 mEq/L
%COHb	1.5%
Hemoglobin	14 gm%

1. The patient is severely hypoxemic as a result of
   a. hypoventilation and venous admixture
   b. hyperventilation causing left shift of the oxygen dissociation curve and reduced SaO_2
   c. increased methemoglobin
   d. ventilation-perfusion imbalance
   e. decreased cardiac output and oxygen transport

2. Arterial oxygen content, in ml O_2/dl, is approximately
   a. 10
   b. 12.5
   c. 14.6
   d. 16
   e. 18

3. $P(A-a)O_2$, in mm Hg, is approximately
   a. 15
   b. 82
   c. 108
   d. 145
   e. 662

4. The patient's acid-base status is best characterized as
   a. marked hyperventilation and metabolic acidosis
   b. respiratory alkalosis and metabolic acidosis
   c. chronic respiratory alkalosis
   d. hyperventilation and acute respiratory alkalosis
   e. respiratory alkalosis and metabolic alkalosis

5. At this point you would treat the patient with
   a. bicarbonate, low-supplemental oxygen (FIO_2 < .40) and antibiotics
   b. 28% oxygen and antibiotics
   c. 40% oxygen by face mask and antibiotics
   d. a mixture of inhaled carbon dioxide and oxygen to lower pH and raise PO_2
   e. 28% oxygen by face mask and blood transfusion to raise oxygen content

Twelve hours later Mr. A appears no better. By this time he is in the intensive care unit and his FIO_2 has been increased to 90% by face mask. However, his PaO_2 is only 55 mm Hg and the chest x-ray now shows extensive bilateral pneumonia. Diagnosis: adult respiratory distress syndrome, most likely from viral pneumonia. Because of oxygenation failure, he is intubated and given artificial ventilation. Settings include 100% inspired oxygen, assist-control ventilator mode at 14 breaths per minute, tidal volume 700 ml. Blood gas results on these settings:

pH	7.40
$PaCO_2$	25 mm Hg
PaO_2	60 mm Hg
SaO_2	85%
HCO_3^-	15 mEq/L
Hemoglobin	13 gm%

6. Now the most likely cause of hypoxemia is
    a. hypoventilation
    b. a change in the position of his O_2 dissociation curve
    c. areas of lung with perfusion but no ventilation
    d. diffusion barrier caused by the pneumonia
    e. not evident from the information provided

7. Arterial oxygen content, in ml O_2/dl blood, is
    a. 12.2
    b. 14.8
    c. 16.4
    d. 17.4
    e. indeterminate

8. $P(A-a)O_2$, in mm Hg, is in the range of
    a. 250-275
    b. 350-375
    c. 400-450
    d. 500-550
    e. over 600

9. Mr. A's acid-base status at this point is best characterized as
   a. chronic metabolic acidosis
   b. chronic respiratory alkalosis
   c. respiratory alkalosis plus metabolic acidosis
   d. metabolic acidosis plus respiratory acidosis
   e. indeterminate from the information provided

10. The best therapeutic approach at this point is to
   a. transfuse one unit of blood
   b. add positive end-expiratory pressure to the ventilator circuit
   c. hyperventilate to shift the O_2-dissociation curve to the left
   d. hypoventilate to shift the O_2-dissociation curve to the right
   e. paralyze the patient in order to provide controlled ventilation

*　*　*

MR. B: A CASE OF CHRONIC OBSTRUCTIVE PULMONARY DISEASE (COPD). Mr. B is a 65-year-old man brought to the emergency department in moderate respiratory distress. He has smoked two packs of cigarettes daily for 45 years and has refused to quit, despite pleading by his family and physician. Pulmonary function tests during past outpatient evaluations showed marked airways obstruction consistent with severe COPD. He was said to be "doing well" until a few days earlier when he developed cough and dyspnea. At that time he reduced his smoking to about half a pack a day.

Examination in the emergency department reveals cyanotic fingers and lips, bilateral wheezing and a few scattered rales in the lung bases. Mr. B's respiratory rate is 30/min and he is using accessory breathing muscles. His feet and legs are edematous and there is a slight hand tremor. Though in some respiratory distress, Mr. B is alert and oriented. His chest x-ray shows flattened diaphragms and hyperinflation consistent with COPD, and no acute infiltrates. Electrocardiogram shows changes consistent with pulmonary hypertension, but no evidence for coronary ischemia.

Mr. B's first set of arterial blood gas data, obtained in the ER while he was breathing room air (FIO_2 .21), shows:

pH	7.36
$PaCO_2$	60 mm Hg
PaO_2	35 mm Hg
SaO_2	51%
HCO_3^-	33 mEq/L
Hemoglobin	17 gm%

1. The most likely explanation for his hypoxemia is
    a. right to left shunting alone
    b. V-Q imbalance alone
    c. hypoventilation and V-Q imbalance
    d. hypoventilation, V-Q imbalance, and increased carbon monoxide level
    e. diffusion block and V-Q imbalance.

2. At this point you would prescribe
    a. 24% FIO_2 by face mask
    b. 50% FIO_2 by face mask
    c. 90% FIO_2 by face mask
    d. artificial ventilation to lower the $PaCO_2$.
    e. phlebotomy of one unit of blood and 100% inspired oxygen

3. Your answer to No. 2 is based on knowledge that
    a. PaO_2 goes up as the $PaCO_2$ goes down
    b. a small PaO_2 change in this part of the oxygen dissociation curve can lead to a relatively large change in SaO_2
    c. in this region of the oxygen dissociation curve, high FIO_2 is needed to improve the SaO_2

    d. hypoxemia is life-threatening, and a patient's PaO_2 should be improved as quickly as possible

    e. removing hemoglobin while adding supplemental oxygen will improve global oxygen transport

Mr. B initially does well on your regimen. However, six hours later he is less alert and falls asleep when not aroused. Repeat arterial blood gas (on supplemental oxygen) reveals

pH	7.10
$PaCO_2$	80 mm Hg
PaO_2	40 mm Hg
SaO_2	64%
HCO_3^-	24 mEq/L

You now conclude that Mr. B requires artificial ventilation because of *altered mental status, hypoventilation, hypoxemia* and *acidemia.*

4. Mr. B's acid-base status before intubation is best characterized as

    a. acute respiratory acidosis

    b. acute respiratory acidosis plus metabolic acidosis

    c. chronic respiratory acidosis plus metabolic acidosis

    d. indeterminate from the information provided

Mr. B is an example of the "blue bloater," a term applied to patients with severe chronic bronchitis who are prone to significant hypoxemia (blue or cyanotic) and right-sided heart failure (bloated or edematous) during exacerbations of their COPD. With good medical management such patients can live for many years. Treatment includes judicious supplemental oxygen, bronchodilators, an occasional course of steroids, and smoking cessation. Potentially lethal are upper respiratory infections, pneumonia, pulmonary embolism and other acute pulmonary insults. Infection was the presumed cause of Mr. B's decompensation.

Mr. B's ventilator is set to deliver 16 breaths/min, tidal volume 800 ml. Blood gas measurements obtained one hour later, on an FIO_2 of 0.40, show

pH	7.30
$PaCO_2$	50 mm Hg
PaO_2	80 mm Hg
SaO_2	90%
HCO_3^-	24 mEq/L
Hemoglobin	16.8 gm%

5. At this point you would
   a. give 50 mEq/L of bicarbonate intravenously and repeat the blood gas
   b. increase FIO_2 to .50
   c. increase tidal volume to 1000 ml
   d. increase breathing frequency to 20/min
   e. not change the ventilator settings

Over the next few days Mr. B is treated with diuretics, steroids, antibiotics and chest physiotherapy, and clinically improves. By the third hospital day his wheezing has cleared and he is alert and feeling better. He points to his endotracheal tube, and indicates through gestures that he wishes it could be removed. At this point the ventilator is set to deliver intermittent mandatory ventilation at six breaths/min, tidal volume 800 ml. His own spontaneous respiratory rate is 10 breaths/min for a total respiratory rate of 16/min. With an FIO_2 of 0.28, he has the following ABG measurements:

pH	7.56
$PaCO_2$	40 mm Hg
PaO_2	65 mm Hg
SaO_2	94%
HCO_3^-	35 mEq/L
Hemoglobin	15 gm%

6. At this point you would
   a. extubate him but maintain the same FIO_2
   b. repeat the blood gas in six hours and, if no worse, extubate him, keeping the same FIO_2
   c. disconnect him from the ventilator without extubation (e.g., using a "blow-by" or "T-piece" at the same FIO_2), so he can breathe spontaneously through the endotracheal tube; repeat the blood gas in a few hours and if the results are adequate, then extubate
   d. remove supplemental oxygen but keep the same ventilator settings and, if his PaO_2 remains adequate, then extubate
   e. decrease the number of IMV breaths per minute while keeping the same FIO_2

7. Your answer to the above question is based on the fact that
   a. there are a number of complications of intubation, and the endotracheal tube should be removed as soon as possible
   b. blood gas measurements reflect the patient's gas exchange status at a particular time and the situation may change rapidly; however, if the blood gas results are essentially the same over a period of time the patient is more likely to remain stable
   c. if a patient can breathe on his own through an endotracheal tube, he will also be able to breathe without one
   d. the patient will be breathing room air after discharge, so you must ensure that his blood gas measurements are at least adequate on room air before extubation
   e. the goal is to achieve his baseline state in terms of gas exchange and not to extubate when blood gas results are better than he can manage without ventilatory assistance

8. Additional information you would like at this time (choose the one best answer)
   a. chest x-ray
   b. P_{50}
   c. %carboxyhemoglobin
   d. serum electrolytes
   e. serum calcium

9. Additional treatment that might be necessary at this point (choose the one best answer)
   a. antibiotics
   b. blood transfusion
   c. increasing FIO_2 to .40
   d. potassium chloride
   e. calcium gluconate

10. Following extubation and after discharge from the hospital Mr. B does well, although he continues to smoke. When at his clinical best after discharge, the most likely set of arterial blood gas values he would manifest on room air is

   a. PaO_2 80; $PaCO_2$ 60; pH 7.35; SaO_2 90
   b. PaO_2 58; $PaCO_2$ 55; pH 7.37; SaO_2 88
   c. PaO_2 90; $PaCO_2$ 35; pH 7.43; SaO_2 90
   d. PaO_2 38; $PaCO_2$ 67; pH 7.38; SaO_2 80
   e. PaO_2 72; $PaCO_2$ 28; pH 7.34; SaO_2 93

* * *

MR. C: A CASE OF INTOXICATION. Mr. C. is a 27-year-old man brought to the emergency room (ER) comatose. He was reportedly found unconscious at home by friends. There is a history of cigarette smoking and a questionable history of drug abuse, but no one stayed around the ER to answer any questions. On examination he is comatose, breathing at 8/min. Vital signs are stable and there is a tachycardia of 100 per minute. ECG confirms sinus tachycardia with no evidence for coronary ischemia. Arterial blood is sent for blood gas analysis (FIO_2 .21) and venous blood is sent for electrolytes and toxicology screen. The arterial blood gas data are first to return and show

pH	7.34
$PaCO_2$	42 mm Hg
PaO_2	82 mm Hg
SaO_2	93% (calculated)
HCO_3^-	22 mEq/L
Hemoglobin	16 gm%

1. What specific information should you obtain at this point? Choose the one best answer.
   a. anion gap
   b. serum K^+
   c. measured oxygen saturation
   d. P_{50}
   e. lactate level

2. The answer to Question 1 is based on the fact that
   a. the anion gap can help determine what type of metabolic acidosis is present
   b. given a metabolic acidosis, it is important to know if hyperkalemia is present, and to what degree
   c. the calculated oxygen saturation could mask a true reduction in SaO_2
   d. the position of the O_2-dissociation curve is an aid to determine if the patient is adequately oxygenated
   e. lactate level might indicate a poor-perfusion state and help diagnose the cause of coma

Additional laboratory tests are ordered and the following results obtained:

SaO_2	50% (measured)
%COHb	47%
lactate	2.0 mMoles/L

Just as you receive these results one of the friends returns to report that Mr. C's cat was found dead in the apartment and that the police and fire department were called. Firemen found carbon monoxide in the apartment air, which they attributed to a faulty space heater. You thank the friend for this belated information and inform him that Mr. C is comatose from acute carbon monoxide intoxication.

3. Mr. C's arterial oxygen content, in ml O_2/dl blood, is approximately
  a. 8.0
  b. 10.9
  b. 11.6
  d. 12.8
  e. indeterminate without more information

4. The position of his oxygen dissociation curve
  a. inhibits unloading of oxygen at the tissue level
  b. inhibits uptake of oxygen at the pulmonary capillary level
  c. is the same as a patient with normal gas exchange whose hemoglobin content is half of Mr. C's
  d. is not clinically relevant in this case
  e. cannot be assessed from the information provided

5. Which of one of the following treatment options would you prescribe at this point?
  a. intubate and give 100% oxygen via a ventilator
  b. intubate and give 60% oxygen via a ventilator
  c. 90% oxygen by face mask
  d. 50% oxygen by face mask
  e. give oxygen via nasal cannula at 3 L/min

A monitor ECG now shows some ischemic cardiac changes, confirmed by a 12-lead ECG. You prescribe intravenous nitroglycerin at a rate of 10 ug/min. He is now receiving 100% inspired oxygen. An hour later arterial blood gas analysis reveals:

pH	7.45
$PaCO_2$	30 mm Hg
PaO_2	525 mm Hg
SaO_2	75%
HCO_3^-	22 mEq/L
%COHb	25%
Hemoglobin	16 gm%

6. How would you interpret these blood gas data?
    a. consistent with improvement from CO intoxication
    b. suggestive of methemoglobinemia
    c. suggestive of aspiration pneumonia
    d. he has developed a metabolic acidosis
    e. he has developed evidence for oxygen toxicity

7. What therapeutic intervention would be most appropriate at this point?
    a. continue FIO_2 at 100%
    b. 1 gm of intravenous methylprednisolone
    c. intravenous methylene blue
    d. 100 mEq sodium bicarbonate delivered intravenously
    e. oxygen therapy in a hyperbaric chamber

The next day, after appropriate therapeutic intervention, Mr. C is awake and alert; he has been extubated and disconnected from the ventilator. At this point arterial blood gas data, on 3 L/min nasal oxygen, show

pH	7.42
$PaCO_2$	36 mm Hg
PaO_2	124 mm Hg
SaO_2	90%
HCO_3^-	24 mEq/L
%COHb	8%
Hemoglobin	15.8 gm%

Mr. C is discharged three days later, in good physical condition. On a return visit, two weeks after discharge, he is asymptomatic. The following blood gases are obtained while he is breathing room air.

pH	7.41
$PaCO_2$	37 mm Hg
PaO_2	88 mm Hg
SaO_2	93%
HCO_3^-	24 mEq/L
%COHb	6%
Hemoglobin	15 gm%

8. What is the most likely reason for the slightly elevated CO level at this point?
      a. he is still exposed to the faulty space heater
      b. he is still smoking cigarettes
      c. he has developed some diffusion block from the acute insult two weeks earlier
      d. has developed ventilation-perfusion imbalance from the acute insult two weeks earlier
      e. the level is consistent with natural occurrence of CO in the body

*　　*　　*

MRS. D: A CASE OF VOMITING AND DEHYDRATION Mrs. D is a 45-year-old alcoholic with several previous hospital admissions for pancreatitis and alcoholic withdrawal symptoms. She presents to the emergency department with a several day history of vomiting and not eating. On examination she is alert and oriented but is also dehydrated and hypotensive, and complaining of mild abdominal pain. Her chest x-ray shows clear lung fields. Initial arterial blood gas (obtained on room air) and serum chemistry values are shown on the next page.

pH	7.47	Na^+	130 mEq/L
$PaCO_2$	48 mm Hg	K^+	2.9 mEq/L
PaO_2	78 mm Hg	Cl^-	77 mEq/L
SaO_2	92%	CO_2	33 mEq/L
HCO_3^-	34 mEq/L		
%COHb	2%	BUN	69 mgm%
Hemoglobin	10 gm%	Creatinine	2.6 mgm%

1. Mrs. D's acid-base status is *best* characterized as
   a. metabolic alkalosis alone
   b. metabolic acidosis alone
   c. metabolic alkalosis *and* metabolic acidosis
   d. metabolic alkalosis *and* compensated respiratory acidosis
   e. compensated respiratory acidosis *and* metabolic acidosis

She is treated with intravenous normal saline and potassium chloride, and nasogastric (NG) suction. Six hours later her arterial blood gas (FIO_2 .21), BUN and electrolyte data show

pH	7.51	Na^+	135 mEq/L
$PaCO_2$	43 mm Hg	K^+	3.2 mEq/L
PaO_2	69 mm Hg	Cl^-	84 mEq/L
SaO_2	91%	CO_2	33 mEq/L
HCO_3^-	33 mEq/L	BUN	58 mgm%

2. All of the following have occurred in the interim, except:
   a. alkalosis has persisted, in part due NG suction
   b. acidosis has improved due to saline infusion
   c. alveolar-arterial PO_2 difference has increased
   d. anion gap has increased
   e. oxygen dissociation curve has shifted to the left

The NG tube is removed and she is given an intravenous dose of acetazolamide, 500 mgm. Saline infusion is continued and supplemental oxygen is given by face mask (FIO_2 31%). Twelve hours later the following arterial blood gas, BUN and electrolyte data are obtained:

pH	7.48	Na^+	137 mEq/L
$PaCO_2$	39 mm Hg	K^+	3.4 mEq/L
PaO_2	95 mm Hg	Cl^-	88 mEq/L
SaO_2	96%	CO_2	29 mEq/L
HCO_3^-	28 mEq/L	BUN	47 mgm%

3. The dose of acetazolamide has apparently
    a. improved oxygenation without elevating $PaCO_2$
    b. increased her serum sodium
    c. caused a slight metabolic acidosis
    d. lowered her anion gap
    e. none of the above

By the next day Mrs. D is better than when admitted. Her blood pressure is normal and the abdominal pain has ceased. She is no longer receiving supplemental oxygen. Arterial blood gases, BUN and electrolyte data now show

pH	7.45	Na^+	139 mEq/L
$PaCO_2$	39 mm Hg	K^+	3.9 mEq/L
PaO_2	79 mm Hg	Cl^-	94 mEq/L
SaO_2	92%	CO_2	28 mEq/L
HCO_3^-	27 mEq/L	BUN	37 mgm%

4. Her acid-base status at this point is best characterized as
    a. normal
    b. mild persistent metabolic acidosis
    c. mild persistent metabolic alkalosis
    d. mild respiratory alkalosis
    e. indeterminate without further information

Mrs. D continues to improve in the hospital and is discharged four days later. No further blood gases are obtained, but serum electrolytes and BUN are obtained daily. Data on the day of discharge:

Na^+	137 mEq/L
K^+	4.2 mEq/L
Cl^-	98 mEq/L
CO_2	22 mEq/L
BUN	20 mgm%

5. These data suggest
   a. normal organ function
   b. persistent metabolic alkalosis
   c. persistent metabolic acidosis
   d. a mild respiratory alkalosis
   e. a mild respiratory acidosis

*   *   *

MR. E: A CASE OF PROLONGED VENTILATOR WEANING.
Mr. E, a 65-year-old man, has been hospitalized two weeks for exacerbation of COPD and acute pneumonia. He was intubated on the day of admission and has since received continuous artificial ventilation. Although he has clinically improved, attempts to wean him from the ventilator have been unsuccessful. He underwent a tracheostomy on hospital day 14. Now his physicians wish to discontinue the indwelling arterial line and to manage his blood gases "non-invasively".

A pulse oximeter is placed on Mr. E's index finger to monitor SaO_2 (SpO_2) and a capnograph is connected to the ventilator circuit to measure end-tidal PCO_2 ($PetCO_2$). Serial blood gases on day 15 are correlated with SpO_2 and $PetCO_2$ data and show the following:

Range of arterial blood gas data on day 15		Range of SpO$_2$ and PetCO$_2$ data on day 15	
FIO$_2$	.40		
pH	7.41 - 7.45		
PaCO$_2$	56 - 63 mm Hg	PetCO$_2$	35 - 40 mm Hg
PaO$_2$	70- 88 mm Hg		
SaO$_2$	90 - 93%	SpO$_2$	89 - 92%
HCO$_3^-$	32 - 36 mEq/L		
%COHb	1.5 - 1.8%		
MetHb	0.8 - 1.0		
Hemoglobin	13.2 - 13.4 gm%		

1. The most likely reason for the large difference between PaCO$_2$ and PetCO$_2$ is
    a. dilution of PetCO$_2$ with room air
    b. dilution of PetCO$_2$ by the high FIO$_2$
    c. the patient's lung disease
    d. the normal spread between the two values
    e. a faulty capnograph

The arterial line is removed and non-invasive measurements are continued. On day 16 they show:

PetCO$_2$	34 mm Hg
SpO$_2$	93%

2. Mr. E. is clinically stable on day 16. All of the following statements are likely true except one. Mr. E
    a. has adequate oxygen content
    b. is hyperventilating
    c. still has a respiratory acidosis
    d. has an increased P(A-a)O$_2$
    e. does not have significant methemoglobinemia

On the afternoon of day 17, the pulse oximeter shows a decline in SpO_2 from 93% to 88% over one hour. The reduction is confirmed with another pulse oximeter. At the same time Mr. E's $PetCO_2$ is steady at 38 mm Hg.

3. All of the following could explain the decline in SpO_2 except
    a. increased V-Q imbalance
    b. reduced PaO_2
    c. carboxyhemoglobin
    d. methemoglobin
    e. right-shift of O_2 dissociation curve

Arterial blood data obtained at this time:

pH	7.44		
$PaCO_2$	60 mm Hg	$PetCO_2$	38 mm Hg
PaO_2	92 mm Hg		
SaO_2	86%	SpO_2	88%
HCO_3^-	36 mEq/L		
%COHb	1.5%		
MetHb	7.8%		
Hemoglobin	13.4 gm%		
FIO_2	0.40		

4. At this point, you should
    a. increase FIO_2
    b. transfuse the patient
    c. review all medications carefully
    d. begin a reducing agent
    e. change the ventilator settings

After making appropriate adjustments, Mr. E's SpO_2 improves. On day 18, his non-invasive measurements and venous CO_2 show:

$PetCO_2$	36 mm Hg
SpO_2	92%
Venous CO_2	33 mEq/L

5. Based on the observed difference between $PaCO_2$ and $PetCO_2$ over the previous two days, Mr. E's arterial pH at this point is approximately

    a. 7.32
    b. 7.37
    c. 7.42
    d. 7.49

These values remain steady over the next several days while settings are adjusted to slowly wean Mr. E off the ventilator. Three weeks into hospitalization, he is receiving only minimal ventilator support (4 breaths/min) and is comfortable. At this time, on an FIO_2 of .35 non-invasive measurements and venous CO_2 show

$PetCO_2$	34 mm Hg
SpO_2	93%
Venous CO_2	36 mEq/L
FIO_2	.30

6. At this point, you wish to disconnect the ventilator and let Mr. E breathe completely on his own. Which of the following is a reasonable method to accomplish this goal?

    a. Insert an arterial line before disconnecting; check blood gas values and, if adequate, disconnect the ventilator; repeat the blood gas one hour later to determine if oxygenation and ventilation are adequate.

    b. Do a single-puncture arterial blood gas prior to disconnecting; if adequate, disconnect ventilator and follow non-invasive measurements and respiratory rate.

    c. Disconnect ventilator; do a single-puncture blood gas one hour after disconnecting to determine if oxygenation and ventilation are adequate.

    d. Disconnect ventilator; follow only the non-invasive measurements and patient's respiratory rate.

Answers to Case Problems

CASE A

1. Answer d:

   The most common cause of hypoxemia is V-Q imbalance: abnormal distribution of ventilation to perfusion among the millions of alveolar-capillary units. Answer a is incorrect because the patient is not hypoventilating; answer b is incorrect because a left-shifted oxygen dissociation curve would give a *higher* SaO_2 at this PaO_2 and in any case would not explain the low PaO_2; answer c is incorrect because there is no reason to suspect methemoglobinemia (SaO_2 is appropriate for this pH and PaO_2). Finally, there is no evidence to support answer e.

2. Answer c:

   $$CaO_2 = SaO_2 \times Hb \ (gm\%) \times 1.34 \ ml \ O_2/gm \ Hb$$

   $$= 0.78 \times 14 \times 1.34$$

   $$= 14.63 \ ml \ O_2/dl \ blood$$

   (Since the PaO_2 is only 38 mm Hg, the dissolved fraction can be ignored.)

3. Answer b:

   $$P(A\text{-}a)O_2 = PAO_2 - PaO_2$$

   $$PAO_2 = FIO_2(P_B - 47 \ mm \ Hg) - 1.2(PaCO_2)$$

   $$= 0.21(760\text{-}47) - 1.2(25) = 120 \ mm \ Hg$$

   $$PaO_2 = 38 \ mm \ Hg$$

   Hence, $P(A\text{-}a)O_2 = 120 - 38 = 82 \ mm \ Hg$

Answers to Case A (continued)

4. Answer d:

    The low $PaCO_2$ indicates that the patient is hyperventilating. The slightly low bicarbonate value is consistent with acute hyperventilation. As there is no evidence for metabolic acidosis, answers a and b are incorrect. Answer c is incorrect because a chronic state would give a lower pH and bicarbonate value. Answer e is incorrect because there is no evidence for metabolic alkalosis.

5. Answer c:

    There is no reason for low-supplemental FIO_2 since the patient is not retaining CO_2. Hence answers a, b, and e are inappropriate. Furthermore, transfusion is not indicated since the patient is not anemic. Answer d is incorrect since this mixture will raise the $PaCO_2$, increase the work of breathing, and do nothing to treat the underlying pneumonia.

6. Answer c:

    The patient has a right-to-left shunt, i.e., some blood is flowing through his lungs that is not being oxygenated. Answer a is incorrect since he is not hypoventilating; answer b is incorrect since changes in the oxygen dissociation curve would not affect the PaO_2; answer d is incorrect since 100% oxygen should overcome a diffusion barrier; finally, answer e is incorrect since shunting *is* evident from the information given. A normal subject breathing 100% oxygen, without significant right-to-left shunting, should have a PaO_2 above 500 mm Hg.

Answers to Case A (continued)

7. Answer b:

   O_2 content = SaO_2 x Hb x 1.34

   = 0.85 x 13 x 1.34

   = 14.81 ml O_2/dl blood

   Since PaO_2 is low (60 mm Hg), the contribution from dissolved oxygen can be ignored.

8. Answer e:

   While breathing 100% oxygen,

   PAO_2 = FIO_2 (PB - 47) - $PaCO_2$

   = 1.0 (713) - 25 = 688 mm Hg

   $P(A\text{-}a)O_2$ = 688 - 60 = 628 mm Hg

   Note that the factor 1.2 in the abbreviated alveolar gas equation becomes 1.00 when breathing 100% oxygen, because nitrogen is fully removed from the lungs (see Chapter 4).

9. Answer c:
   Neither acid-base disorder alone (respiratory alkalosis, metabolic acidosis) would give a pH of 7.40. When combined in the same patient, the two disorders can mask their respective pH changes (low for acidosis, high for alkalosis) and result in a normal pH. Note that the patient is hyperventilating more than expected for this degree of metabolic acidosis and thus has a primary respiratory alkalosis, caused by hypoxemia, pneumonia, and the artificial ventilation.

Answers to Case A (continued)

10. Answer b:

    There is no compelling reason to transfuse this patient since his hemoglobin content is near normal. As to answers c and d, the patient has a normal pH and any shift of the curve by altering pH can have an unpredictable and adverse effect on the patient. Paralysis is sometimes used in patients who cannot be adequately ventilated, but his $PaCO_2$ is already low. The best answer of the choices given is to add positive end-expiratory pressure (PEEP), a technique that allows better oxygen transfer at the same FIO_2.

CASE B

1. Answer d:

    First, the patient is hypoventilating ($PaCO_2$ is 60 mm Hg), providing at least one reason for the reduced PaO_2. Second, assuming barometric pressure of 760 mm Hg, $P(A-a)O_2$ is 37 mm Hg, which is an elevated value breathing room air and indicates ventilation-perfusion imbalance, most likely due to his COPD. Finally, note that a PaO_2 of 35 mm Hg should give an SaO_2 over 60% (pH 7.36), not 51%. The lower-than-expected SaO_2 indicates "something else" must be binding to the patient's hemoglobin besides oxygen. In a heavy smoker, excess carbon monoxide is the most likely explanation.

    Despite the elevated hemoglobin content this patient's arterial oxygen content is reduced to about 11.8 ml O_2/dl. He is thus hypoxemic for three reasons: hypoventilation, ventilation-perfusion imbalance, and excess blood carbon monoxide.

Answers to Case B (continued)

2. Answer a:

  This patient is a CO_2 retainer; providing too high an FIO_2 runs the risk of blunting any hypoxic drive to breathe and causing further hypoventilation. Thus low supplemental FIO_2 (e.g., 24%) is the optimal initial treatment.

3. Answer b:

  A review of the oxygen dissociation curve shows that the patient's PaO_2 is on the so-called steep part of the curve. Hence, a small increment in the PaO_2 will lead to a relatively large increment in SaO_2 (when compared with the flat parts of the oxygen dissociation curve). As a result, oxygen content can increase without cutting off the hypoxic drive to breathe.

4. Answer b:

  If his only acid-base problem was acute respiratory acidosis, HCO_3^- should be higher than 24 mEq/L (pH at this $PaCO_2$ would be about 7.15, not 7.10.) Since his pH and HCO_3^- are lower than predicted for acute respiratory acidosis, he must have another condition contributing to low pH, i.e., metabolic acidosis.

5. Answer e:

  After one hour of artificial ventilation, the patient's $PaCO_2$ has decreased from 80 mm Hg to 50 mm Hg. The patient is in a transient situation and has not reached a steady state in terms of ventilation. Another hour may show further reduction of his $PaCO_2$. Thus it is best to leave the ventilator settings alone and especially to do nothing that will lower the $PaCO_2$ any faster (as may occur from the steps in answers c and d). The step in answer a is unnecessary since the pH is increasing from reduction of $PaCO_2$; extra HCO_3^- may actually cause an unwanted alkalosis as $PaCO_2$ decreases further.

Answers to Case B (continued)

5. (continued)

The step in answer b is unwarranted for two reasons: his PaO_2 is adequate while breathing 40% inspired oxygen, and SaO_2 will increase as his pH increases (O_2-dissociation curve shifts to left).

6. Answer e or c. See answer to Question 7.

7. Answer e:

Your goal should be to return the patient's acid-base and ventilatory status close to what it will be while breathing room air, off the ventilator. He now has a metabolic alkalosis, caused by the diuretics and steroids, and manifested by high pH and normal $PaCO_2$ (with resulting high HCO_3^-). The compensation for metabolic alkalosis is hypoventilation; once the patient is extubated, hypoventilation may occur rapidly, at least partly to compensate the alkalosis. Another reason the patient may hypoventilate once extubated relates to his chronic lung disease. Based on his history and presenting arterial blood gas values, he is most likely a chronic carbon dioxide retainer.

One danger of sudden hypoventilation is the rapid fall that can occur in PaO_2 as $PaCO_2$ increases. Optimally one should: 1) allow the patient to achieve his baseline state of hypoventilation while being artificially ventilated so he does not acutely hypoventilate once extubated; and 2) remove any metabolic cause of further hypoventilation by aggressively treating the metabolic alkalosis. One approach is to decrease the number of IMV breaths/min while correcting the alkalosis. In this way, the patient can gradually hypoventilate while acid-base and oxygen status are closely monitored. Another 24 hours of such management might assure a more successful extubation.

Answers to Case B (continued)

7. (continued)

There are many approaches to weaning such patients from the ventilator; of the answers provided here, e seems best for the reasons given above. However, other physicians might opt for answer c, another reasonable approach. In managing such cases, it is more important to be aware of the physiologic principles involved and of the clinical response to treatment than to follow rigid rules.

8. Answer d:

Since the patient has metabolic alkalosis, you want to evaluate his serum K^+; none of the other tests seem particularly indicated at this time.

9. Answer d:

Most likely the patient is hypokalemic because of the diuretic therapy.

10. Answer b:

Answer a is incorrect since the patient would not have a PaO_2 of 80 mm Hg with a $PaCO_2$ of 60 mm Hg; such values would constitute a negative $P(A-a)O_2$. Answer c is unlikely since we know he is a chronic CO_2 retainer; these blood gas measurements show a slightly reduced $PaCO_2$ and a normal PaO_2, values unlikely in a patient with such severe respiratory disease. Answer d is unlikely since the PaO_2 is too low for him to be "doing well." On a physiologic basis, this PaO_2 would give an SaO_2 less than 75%, not one of 80%. Answer e is unlikely since these blood gas values suggest a metabolic acidosis, which he has no reason to have. Also, it is unlikely he could hyperventilate to this degree and considered to be "doing well."

CASE C

1. Answer c:

    The calculated SaO_2 may be inaccurate if the position of the oxygen dissociation curve is shifted from normal. The P_{50} would give you this information but it is a much more complex test to run than is the SaO_2. The other information could be useful but SaO_2 measurement should be obtained first in this case.

2. Answer c: see explanation above.

3. Answer b:

    $$CaO_2 = (SaO_2 \text{ x Hb x } 1.34) + (.003 \text{ x } 82)$$

    $$= (0.50 \text{ x } 16 \text{ x } 1.34) + .25$$

    $$= 10.97 \text{ ml } O_2/dl$$

    Note that the answer is b with or without calculation of the dissolved oxygen fraction.

4. Answer a:

    His oxygen dissociation curve is shifted to the left and thus unloading of oxygen is retarded at the tissue level.

5. Answer a:

    This patient is comatose and critically hypoxemic. Of the options listed, the best is to intubate him and give 100% oxygen via ventilator. A hyperbaric chamber would also be appropriate but such a device is available in only a small minority of hospitals.

6. Answer a:

    These results are entirely consistent with improvement from CO intoxication; his SaO_2 remains low but is rising as CO is removed from the blood. Because the patient

Answers to Case C (continued)

6. (continued)
> is receiving nitroglycerin, he is at some risk for developing methemoglobinemia. However, the SaO_2 + %COHb total 100%, so there is no evidence for methemoglobin. His PaO_2 is appropriate for someone receiving 100% oxygen, so there is also no reason to suspect aspiration pneumonia. His blood gases do not suggest a metabolic acidosis. Finally, it is too soon to develop oxygen toxicity.

7. Answer a or e:
> There is no indication for the other three maneuvers. You want to keep the FIO_2 high to eliminate carbon monoxide quickly, and it is too soon to worry about oxygen toxicity. Facilities with a hyperbaric chamber would probably opt for that form of therapy, since some studies suggest better long term results when CO intoxication is treated with hyperbaric oxygen. However, hyperbaric chambers are not available in most hospitals.

8. Answer b:
> Mr. C became comatose from a very high CO level. The level is now only 6%, slightly elevated and most consistent with cigarette smoking. Neither diffusion block nor V-Q imbalance would cause an elevated CO; the CO level from natural breakdown of heme is less than 3%.

CASE D

1. Answer c:
> She has an elevated anion gap and an elevated bicarbonate. The anion gap acidosis can be attributed to dehydration with poor perfusion, and perhaps some mild

Answers to Case D (continued)

1. (continued)
    renal insufficiency, although the elevated BUN and creatinine could all be due to dehydration. The metabolic alkalosis is due to vomiting and consequent hypokalemia. The CO_2 retention could be solely a compensation for metabolic alkalosis.

2. Answer d:
    Her anion gap has actually decreased with volume infusion.

3. Answer c:
    The dose of acetazolamide has induced a mild metabolic acidosis, lowering the bicarbonate.

4. Answer b:
    Her anion gap is still elevated at 17 mEq/L, suggesting a mild persistent metabolic acidosis.

5. Answer c:
    These data suggest she has persistent metabolic acidosis, probably from underlying mild renal insufficiency.

CASE E

1. Answer c:
    The patient has increased dead space from lung disease and for this reason manifests a large ($PaCO_2$ - $PetCO_2$). (The normal difference is minimal, 0 to a few mm Hg). Answers a and e are also possible, and the capnograph and its connections should be frequently checked. FIO_2 has no direct effect on $PaCO_2$ or end-tidal PCO_2.

Answers to Case E (continued)

2. Answer b:

    The initial spread between $PaCO_2$ and $PetCO_2$ was 21-23 mm Hg. There is no reason to expect any change in this difference, so the patient's $PaCO_2$ is still high; he is not hyperventilating. The other answers are correct.

3. Answer c:

    Carboxyhemoglobin is not measured by pulse oximeters but is "read" as oxyhemoglobin. Thus an elevation in COHb is not reflected in SpO_2. All the other conditions could lead to a true reduction in SaO_2 and SpO_2.

4. Answer c:

    This patient now has an increased methemoglobin level. He was receiving acetaminophen (Tylenol), a drug sometimes associated with increased methemoglobin. The drug was discontinued. None of the other steps listed are particularly indicated at this time.

5. Answer b:

    You can use the Henderson-Hasselbalch equation or the acid-base map in Figure 6-2. Either way, you need HCO_3^- and $PaCO_2$. For the former, use the total CO_2 of 33 mEq/L. For $PaCO_2$, add the $PaCO_2$ - $PetCO_2$ difference (about 22 mEq/L) to the most recent $PetCO_2$ measurement (36 mEq/L) to obtain an estimated $PaCO_2$ of 58 mm Hg. These values translate into a pH of 7.37.

6. Answer d:

    There is no compelling reason to resume measurement of arterial blood gases. Respiratory rate is a good monitor of clinical distress and, with SpO_2 and $PetCO_2$, should provide enough information to monitor the patient once he is disconnected from the ventilator. If he develops any respiratory distress, he can be quickly reconnected and blood gases can then be measured.

CHAPTER 8.

Putting It All Together: Free Text Interpretations

In this chapter are 20 brief clinical descriptions along with blood gas data. In some cases electrolyte data are also provided. Base excess is omitted for most of the data sets since it is not always provided with blood gas reports; also, you should learn to interpret acid-base status without it (see page 105).

Interpret all the blood gas data for each case in terms of VENTILATION, OXYGENATION and ACID-BASE STATUS. Do those calculations appropriate for your interpretations. Assume barometric pressure is 760 mm Hg.

The specific wording of the interpretations is up to you. Adopt the role of consultant. Assume another student or physician has just presented the data to you and has asked for your formal interpretation. Make sure you *WRITE DOWN YOUR INTERPRETATIONS BEFORE CHECKING THE ANSWER SECTION.* If you make a "mental interpretation only," you will be cheating yourself of a valuable learning exercise.

Do one or two sets, compare your interpretations with those provided at the end of the chapter, then go back and do some more. I recommend that you not try to complete all 20 cases in one sitting.

1. A 55-year-old man is evaluated in the pulmonary lab for shortness of breath. His regular medications include a diuretic for hypertension and one aspirin a day. He smokes a pack of cigarettes a day.

FIO$_2$ .21
pH   7.53
PaCO$_2$ 37 mm Hg
PaO$_2$ 62 mm Hg
SaO$_2$ 87%
HCO$_3^-$ 30 mEq/L
%COHb   7.8%
%MetHb   0.8%
Hb   14 gm%
CaO$_2$ 16.5 ml O$_2$/dl

OXYGENATION:

VENTILATION:

ACID-BASE:

2. A 23-year-old woman is seen in the emergency department for difficulty in breathing. Her lung exam and chest x-ray are normal.

FIO$_2$ .21   Na$^+$ 141 mEq/L
pH   7.55   K$^+$ 4.1 mEq/L
PaCO$_2$ 25 mm Hg   Cl$^-$ 106 mEq/L
PaO$_2$ 112 mm Hg   CO$_2$ 24 mEq/L
SaO$_2$ 98%
HCO$_3^-$ 21 mEq/L
%COHb   1.8%
%MetHb   0.6%
Hb   13 gm%
CaO$_2$ 17.4 ml O$_2$/dl

OXYGENATION:

VENTILATION:

ACID-BASE:

3. An 60-year-old woman is in the coronary care unit for evaluation of chest pain. She is receiving supplemental oxygen by face mask and her chest x-ray shows pulmonary edema.

FIO_2	.40
pH	7.22
$PaCO_2$	38 mm Hg
PaO_2	76 mm Hg
SaO_2	84%
HCO_3^-	15 mEq/L
%COHb	2.2%
%MetHb	6.2%
Hb	10.8 gm%
CaO_2	12.2 ml O_2/dl

OXYGENATION:

VENTILATION:

ACID-BASE:

4. A 46-year-old man has been in the hospital two days, with pneumonia. He was recovering but has just become diaphoretic, dyspneic and hypotensive.

FIO_2	3 L/min nasal oxygen
pH	7.40
$PaCO_2$	20 mm Hg
PaO_2	80 mm Hg
SaO_2	95%
HCO_3^-	12 mEq/L
%COHb	1.0%
%MetHb	0.2%
Hb	13.3 gm%
CaO_2	17.2 ml O_2/dl

OXYGENATION:

VENTILATION:

ACID-BASE:

5. A 35-year-old man is in the pulmonary lab for evaluation of dyspnea.

FIO_2	.21
pH	7.43
$PaCO_2$	37 mm Hg
PaO_2	92 mm Hg
SaO_2	96%
HCO_3^-	24 mEq/L
%COHb	1.5%
%MetHb	0.6%
Hb	14.8 gm%
CaO_2	19.3 ml O_2/dl

OXYGENATION:

VENTILATION:

ACID-BASE:

6. A 44-year-old comatose man is brought to the emergency department. His blood pressure and heart rate are normal.

FIO_2	.40	Na^+	136 mEq/L
pH	7.46	K^+	3.8 mEq/L
$PaCO_2$	25 mm Hg	Cl^-	101 mEq/L
PaO_2	232 mm Hg	CO_2	15 mEq/L
SaO_2	55%		

HCO$_3^-$	17 mEq/L
%COHb	43%
%MetHb	1.2%
Hb	13.7 gm%
CaO$_2$	10.8 ml O$_2$/dl

OXYGENATION:

VENTILATION:

ACID-BASE:

7. A 30-year-old woman is being evaluated in the emergency department for chest pain of sudden onset.

FIO$_2$	.21
pH	7.50
PaCO$_2$	30 mm Hg
PaO$_2$	85 mm Hg
SaO$_2$	95%
HCO$_3^-$	23 mEq/L
%COHb	1.3%
%MetHb	0.3%
Hb	12 gm%
CaO$_2$	15.5 ml O$_2$/dl

OXYGENATION:

VENTILATION:

ACID-BASE:

8. A 23-year-old woman is brought in a lethargic state to the emergency room. She has a history of diabetes.

FIO_2	.21
pH	7.02
$PaCO_2$	12 mm Hg
PaO_2	115 mm Hg
SaO_2	93%
HCO_3^-	3 mEq/L
%COHb	1.1%
%MetHb	0.1%
Hb	12.2 gm%
CaO_2	15.2 ml O_2/dl

OXYGENATION:

VENTILATION:

ACID-BASE:

9. A 39-year-old man is being evaluated in the outpatient department for a nervous condition. He is noticeably anxious and shaking, and has a history of alcoholism.

FIO_2	.21
pH	7.54
$PaCO_2$	54 mm Hg
PaO_2	65 mm Hg
SaO_2	97%
HCO_3^-	34 mEq/L
%COHb	1.1%
%MetHb	0.4%
Hb	8 gm%
CaO_2	10.6 ml O_2/dl

OXYGENATION:

VENTILATION:

ACID-BASE:

10. A 58-year-old woman is brought to the emergency room after she vomited bright red blood. She is mildly hypotensive and tachypneic, breathing 36 times a minute.

FIO_2	.21
pH	7.34
$PaCO_2$	35 mm Hg
PaO_2	69 mm Hg
SaO_2	88%
HCO_3^-	20 mEq/L
%COHb	6.1%
%MetHb	0.4%
Hb	4 gm%
CaO_2	4.92 ml O_2/dl

OXYGENATION:

VENTILATION:

ACID-BASE:

11. A 48-year-old man is being evaluated in the emergency department for acute dyspnea.

FIO_2	.21
pH	7.19
$PaCO_2$	65 mm Hg
PaO_2	45 mm Hg
SaO_2	90%
HCO_3^-	24 mEq/L
%COHb	1.1%
%MetHb	0.4
Hb	15.1 gm%
CaO_2	18.3 ml O_2/dl

OXYGENATION:

VENTILATION:

ACID-BASE:

12. A 65-year-old woman has become suddenly hypotensive one day following surgery for a fractured femur.

FIO_2	.21
pH	7.47
$PaCO_2$	32 mm Hg
PaO_2	57 mm Hg
SaO_2	83%
HCO_3^-	23 mEq/L
%COHb	2.1%
%MetHb	0.5%
Hb	11.5 gm%
CaO_2	12.9 ml O_2/dl

Her arterial blood gas prior to surgery (on room air): PaO_2 84 mm Hg, $PaCO_2$ 39 mm Hg.

OXYGENATION:

VENTILATION:

ACID-BASE:

13. The following arterial blood gas data were obtained during a cardiopulmonary resuscitation.

FIO_2	1.00 (via manual bagging)
pH	7.10

PaCO$_2$	76 mm Hg
PaO$_2$	125 mm Hg
SaO$_2$	99%
HCO$_3^-$	20 mEq/L
%COHb	2.1%
%MetHb	0.5%
Hb	12 gm%
CaO$_2$	16.3 ml O$_2$/dl

OXYGENATION:

VENTILATION:

ACID-BASE:

14. An 28-year-old woman is in the emergency department following an attempted suicide with aspirin.

FIO$_2$	.40	Na$^+$	140 mEq/L
pH	7.35	K$^+$	4.1 mEq/L
PaCO$_2$	16 mm Hg	Cl$^-$	100 mEq/L
PaO$_2$	130 mm Hg	CO$_2$	16 mEq/L
SaO$_2$	98%		
HCO$_3^-$	15 mEq/L		
%COHb	1.1%		
%MetHb	0.5%		
Hb	12.6 gm%		
CaO$_2$	16.9 ml O$_2$/dl		

OXYGENATION:

VENTILATION:

ACID-BASE:

15. An 65-year-old man is evaluated for marked obesity and hypertension in the outpatient clinic. His chief complaint is shortness of breath on exertion.

FIO_2	.21
pH	7.33
$PaCO_2$	59 mm Hg
PaO_2	54 mm Hg
SaO_2	89%
HCO_3^-	30 mEq/L
%COHb	4.1%
%MetHb	0.5%
Hb	18 gm%
CaO_2	21.6 ml O_2/dl

OXYGENATION:

VENTILATION:

ACID-BASE:

16. Shortly after gastrointestinal endoscopy, a 55-year-old man is noted to increase his respiratory rate and turn blue. Before endoscopy, his room air blood gas was normal.

FIO_2	.21
pH	7.34
$PaCO_2$	31 mm Hg
PaO_2	79 mm Hg
SaO_2	75%
HCO_3^-	16 mEq/L
%COHb	1.1%
%MetHb	18%
Hb	11.1 gm%
CaO_2	11.4 ml O_2/dl

OXYGENATION:

VENTILATION:

ACID-BASE:

17. A 70-year-old man is intubated for respiratory failure; the ventilator settings include tidal volume 700 ml, and assist-control mode at 14 breaths/min.

FIO_2	.40
pH	7.34
$PaCO_2$	48 mm Hg
PaO_2	80 mm Hg
SaO_2	95%
HCO_3^-	25 mEq/L
%COHb	2.1%
%MetHb	1.1%
Hb	14.5 gm%
CaO_2	18.7 ml O_2/dl

OXYGENATION:

VENTILATION:

ACID-BASE:

18. A 23-year-old man is being evaluated in the emergency room for severe pneumonia. His respiratory rate is 38/min and he is using his accessory breathing muscles.

FIO_2	.90	Na^+	145 mEq/L
pH	7.29	K^+	4.1 mEq/L
$PaCO_2$	55 mm Hg	Cl^-	100 mEq/L
PaO_2	47 mm Hg	CO_2	24 mEq/L

SaO_2	86%
HCO_3^-	23 mEq/L
%COHb	2.1%
%MetHb	1.1%
Hb	13 gm%
CaO_2	15.8 ml O_2/dl

OXYGENATION:

VENTILATION:

ACID-BASE:

19.   An arterial blood gas is obtained before and during a treadmill exercise test in a 39-year-old man without any known respiratory problem. (RR = respiratory rate/min)

	Before exercise	During exercise
RR	12	30
FIO_2	.21	.21
pH	7.43	7.41
$PaCO_2$	39	37 mm Hg
PaO_2	96	88 mm Hg
SaO_2	95	95%
HCO_3^-	24	24 mEq/L

OXYGENATION:

VENTILATION:

ACID-BASE:

20. An arterial blood gas is obtained before and during a treadmill exercise test in a 55-year-old man with severe COPD.

	Before exercise	During exercise
RR	12	40
FIO_2	.21	.21
pH	7.38	7.32
$PaCO_2$	42	51 mm Hg
PaO_2	72	55 mm Hg
SaO_2	92	83%
HCO_3^-	24	25 mEq/L

OXYGENATION:

VENTILATION:

ACID-BASE:

Free Text Interpretations of Blood Gas Data

1.

OXYGENATION: The PaO_2 and SaO_2 are both reduced on room air. The $P(A-a)O_2$ is elevated (approximately 43 mm Hg), so the low PaO_2 can be attributed to V-Q imbalance, i.e., a pulmonary problem. SaO_2 is reduced, in part from the low PaO_2 but mainly from elevated carboxyhemoglobin, which in turn can be attributed to cigarettes. The arterial oxygen content is adequate.

VENTILATION: Adequate for the patient's level of CO_2 production; the patient is neither hyper- nor hypoventilating.

ACID-BASE: Elevated pH and HCO_3^- suggest a state of metabolic alkalosis, most likely related to the patient's diuretic; his serum K^+ should be checked to look for hypokalemia.

2.

OXYGENATION: The PaO_2 is normal on room air for this degree of hyperventilation, and her oxygen content is adequate.

VENTILATION: She is hyperventilating.

ACID-BASE: High pH and low $PaCO_2$ are consistent with acute respiratory alkalosis. The slightly low HCO_3^- is expected solely from acute hyperventilation and does not signify a metabolic acidosis. In line with this, her serum electrolytes are normal and there is no elevation of the anion gap.

3.

OXYGENATION: The $P(A-a)O_2$ is elevated on 40% oxygen, consistent with V-Q imbalance from pulmonary edema. SaO_2 is reduced because of a rightward shift of the oxygen dissociation curve (due to acidemia) and an elevated methemoglobin. The elevated methemoglobin may be related to drug therapy. Is she on nitrates? Her oxygen content is reduced from both low SaO_2 and anemia.

VENTILATION: The patient has normal alveolar ventilation, which seems clinically inappropriate in view of her apparent metabolic acidosis.

Free Text Interpretations (continued)

3. (continued)
ACID-BASE: Low pH and normal $PaCO_2$ suggest severe metabolic acidosis with inadequate respiratory compensation; the patient is at risk for developing hypercapnia and respiratory failure.

4.
OXYGENATION: The PaO_2 is lower than expected for someone hyperventilating to this degree and receiving supplemental oxygen, and points to significant V-Q imbalance. The oxygen content is adequate.
VENTILATION: $PaCO_2$ is half normal and indicates marked hyperventilation.
ACID-BASE: Normal pH with very low bicarbonate and $PaCO_2$ indicates combined respiratory alkalosis and metabolic acidosis. If these changes are of sudden onset the diagnosis of sepsis should be strongly considered, especially in someone with a documented infection.

5.
OXYGENATION: PaO_2 and SaO_2 are within normal limits; there is no evidence for resting hypoxemia.
VENTILATION: Within normal limits.
ACID-BASE: Within normal limits.
    In summary, these are normal resting arterial blood gases.

6.
OXYGENATION: The PaO_2 is increased appropriately for 40% inspired oxygen, suggesting no significant V-Q imbalance. However, the patient's SaO_2 is markedly reduced due to a carboxyhemoglobin level of 43%. As a result, the oxygen content is reduced. Oxygen delivery in this patient may be markedly compromised because of alkalemia and elevated CO, both factors that shift the oxygen dissociation curve to the left (i.e., cause hemoglobin to hold oxygen more tightly than normal).

Free Text Interpretations (continued)

6. (continued)

VENTILATION: The patient is hyperventilating.

ACID-BASE: Slightly elevated pH with low $PaCO_2$ and low bicarbonate could represent either a) chronic respiratory alkalosis, or b) respiratory alkalosis plus metabolic acidosis. Since the patient's anion gap is elevated (20 mEq/L), b) is more likely.

7.

OXYGENATION: The PaO_2 is adequate, but the $P(A-a)O_2$ is increased (approximately 29 mm Hg), indicating V-Q imbalance. The symptom of chest pain suggests pulmonary embolism as a possible diagnosis. The oxygen content is adequate.

VENTILATION: Hyperventilation.

ACID-BASE: Consistent with acute respiratory alkalosis.

8.

OXYGENATION: The PaO_2 is appropriately increased above normal due to extreme hyperventilation. SaO_2 is slightly reduced for this PaO_2 (due to a rightward shift of the oxygen dissociation curve from acidemia) but is nonetheless adequate, as is the patient's oxygen content.

VENTILATION: $PaCO_2$ is very low, indicating extreme hyperventilation. This $PaCO_2$, which is at or near the limit for voluntary hyperventilation, is the expected response for severe metabolic acidosis.

ACID-BASE: pH and $PaCO_2$ are consistent with a state of severe diabetic ketoacidosis.

9.

OXYGENATION: PaO_2 is reduced but the SaO_2 is normal due to leftward shift of the oxygen dissociation curve. The patient is markedly anemic and as a result his oxygen content is reduced.

VENTILATION: The patient is hypoventilating.

ACID-BASE: Elevated pH and $PaCO_2$ suggest both metabolic alkalosis and respiratory acidosis. Suggest checking the patient's serum potassium.

Free Text Interpretations (continued)

10.

OXYGENATION: The PaO_2 is reduced on room air, indicating V-Q imbalance. Her SaO_2 is further reduced from an elevated carbon monoxide level. Finally, oxygen content is markedly reduced, in part due to low SaO_2 but mainly because of severe anemia.

VENTILATION: $PaCO_2$ is low-normal but may reflect mild hyperventilation due to metabolic acidosis.

ACID-BASE: The pH and $PaCO_2$ are suggestive of a mild metabolic acidosis, most likely related to the patient's hypotension and hypoxemia (low oxygen content).

11.

OXYGENATION: The patient's PaO_2 is reduced for two reasons: hypercapnia and V-Q imbalance, the latter apparent from an elevated $P(A-a)O_2$ (approximately 27 mm Hg).

VENTILATION: The patient is hypoventilating.

ACID-BASE: pH and $PaCO_2$ are suggestive of acute respiratory acidosis plus metabolic acidosis; the calculated HCO_3^- is lower than expected from acute respiratory acidosis alone.

12.

OXYGENATION: The PaO_2 is very low on room air, due to V-Q imbalance. Given her prior normal PaO_2, an acute pulmonary event has occurred. Considering her post-operative status the most likely diagnosis is acute pulmonary embolism and a lung scan is clearly indicated. In addition, her oxygen content is slightly reduced, from both low SaO_2 and anemia.

VENTILATION: She is hyperventilating.

ACID-BASE: High pH and low $PaCO_2$ are consistent with acute uncomplicated respiratory alkalosis.

Free Text Interpretations (continued)

13.
OXYGENATION: On 100% oxygen via Ambu bag, the patient has a large $P(A-a)O_2$, indicating significant right to left shunting. Oxygen content was adequate at the time the blood gas was obtained.
VENTILATION: The patient is not being adequately ventilated by the Ambu bag.
ACID-BASE: This pH and $PaCO_2$ indicate acute respiratory acidosis plus metabolic acidosis; acute hypoventilation to a $PaCO_2$ of 76 mm Hg alone would lead to a pH higher than 7.10 and a HCO_3^- higher than 20 mEq/L.

14.
OXYGENATION: The PaO_2 is adequate but reduced for this FIO_2, indicating a state of V-Q imbalance. With an overdose situation one should consider, among other possibilities, aspiration pneumonia. The oxygen content is adequate.
VENTILATION: The patient is markedly hyperventilating.
ACID-BASE: pH and $PaCO_2$ are consistent with combined respiratory alkalosis and metabolic acidosis, a state often seen in aspirin overdose. The anion gap is elevated at 24 mEq/L, also indicating metabolic acidosis.

15.
OXYGENATION: This patient has a low PaO_2 for two reasons: V-Q imbalance (apparent from elevated $P(A-a)O_2$) and hypercapnia. His oxygen content is adequate only because of polycythemia, which in turn is most likely related to chronically low PaO_2.
VENTILATION: The patient is hypoventilating, perhaps related to obesity.
ACID-BASE: Consistent with partially compensated respiratory acidosis.

Free Text Interpretations (continued)

16.
OXYGENATION: The patient's PaO_2 is slightly low, but his SaO_2 is much lower than expected for this PaO_2, due to an elevated methemoglobin level; this in turn is most likely related to reaction from local anesthetic used during the procedure (e.g., benzocaine). His oxygen content is low from both low SaO_2 and anemia.
VENTILATION: He is hyperventilating.
ACID-BASE: This patient has developed a mild metabolic acidosis, most likely related to sudden onset of hypoxemia.

17.
OXYGENATION: This patient's PaO_2 is adequate but much lower than expected for an FIO_2 of .40, indicating significant V-Q imbalance. His SaO_2 and oxygen content are adequate.
VENTILATION: The patient is being slightly hypoventilated by the ventilator.
ACID-BASE: This pH and $PaCO_2$ suggest mild acute respiratory acidosis. The ventilator settings should be increased to improve alveolar ventilation, lower $PaCO_2$ and increase pH.

18.
OXYGENATION: The PaO_2 and SaO_2 are both markedly reduced on 90% inspired oxygen.
VENTILATION: The patient is hypoventilating despite the presence of tachypnea, indicating significant dead space ventilation. This is a dangerous situation that suggests the need for artificial ventilation.
ACID-BASE: The low pH, high $PaCO_2$ and slightly low HCO_3^- point to combined acute respiratory acidosis and metabolic acidosis.

Free Text Interpretations (continued)

19.

OXYGENATION: The PaO_2 and SaO_2 are normal both before and during exercise; there is no oxygen desaturation with this level of exercise.

VENTILATION: Normal alveolar ventilation before treadmill exercise. During exercise, alveolar ventilation remains adequate for the increase in CO_2 production.

ACID-BASE: Normal before and during exercise.

In summary, this is a normal blood gas response to submaximal exercise; neither the PaO_2 nor the $PaCO_2$ change significantly.

20.

OXYGENATION: Before exercise, PaO_2 and SaO_2 are slightly reduced on room air. During exercise, the PaO_2 falls significantly, possibly reflecting diffusion impairment from the patient's COPD.

VENTILATION: Normal alveolar ventilation before exercise. During exercise, $PaCO_2$ increases, reflecting inadequate alveolar ventilation for the increase in CO_2 production that accompanies exercise.

ACID-BASE: Normal before exercise. During exercise, the patient becomes hypercapnic from inadequate alveolar ventilation, and develops acute respiratory acidosis.

CHAPTER 9.

Pitfalls in Blood Gas Interpretation

As with any lab result, there are potential pitfalls in interpreting blood gas data. This chapter briefly discusses the most common pitfalls, which span the range from sampling errors to ignoring valid data. It is beyond the scope of this book to present techniques of drawing and analyzing the arterial blood sample, but these aspects should be recognized as the source of potential errors in interpretation. Several excellent texts cover technical and methodologic aspects in detail and I recommend them to interested readers in the Bibliography. Common pitfalls that could affect interpretation include the following:

1. **NOT AN ARTERIAL SAMPLE.** Sometimes there is no way to know if blood gas data are from an arterial or venous blood sample. The person drawing the sample can usually tell the difference. If blood pulsates into the syringe and the syringe plunger rises on its own, the sample is most likely arterial; venous pressure is seldom sufficient to fill a syringe. Conversely, if the syringe can only be filled by manually pulling on the plunger *and* the PaO_2 is very low, the sample is likely venous. Peripheral vein PO_2 is almost always less than 40 mm Hg, and often less than 30 mm Hg. A $PO_2 > 40$ mm Hg or oxygen saturation $> 75\%$ is most likely *not* from a pure venous sample. Unlike venous PO_2 and O_2 saturation, venous pH and PCO_2 are often close to arterial values, so abnormal pH and PCO_2 cannot be used to classify any blood gas data as venous in origin.

On occasion there is venous admixture; the sample contains *some* venous blood and therefore a lower PO_2 than would be found in pure arterial blood. Venous admixture is more likely to occur with multiple passes of the syringe needle, and also when the femoral artery is sampled; this artery is adjacent to the large capacity femoral vein. A single puncture with rapid filling helps ensure against sample contamination. When in doubt about the validity of a blood sample, the test should be repeated or a pulse oximetry measurement obtained instead.

2. **PATIENT NOT IN A STEADY STATE.** Before blood gas data are used for patient management, the patient should be in a steady state in terms of oxygenation and ventilation. This pitfall can occur if the blood sample is from a patient recently a) connected to an artificial ventilator, or b) changed to a different FIO_2. It takes only about three minutes for people with healthy lungs to achieve a steady state on supplemental oxygen; patients with chronic airways obstruction may take up to 20 minutes to reach a steady state. As a general rule, wait at least 20 minutes before drawing a blood sample if there has been a change in FIO_2. In artificially-ventilated patients, where both $PaCO_2$ and PaO_2 may be affected after a change in ventilator settings, wait at least a half hour for the patient to reach a steady state.

3. **SAMPLE SYRINGE CONTAINS TOO MUCH ANTI-COAGULANT.** Several studies have analyzed the effects of anticoagulant on blood gas data. The effect depends on the type of anticoagulant (most commonly lithium heparin; sometimes sodium heparin), its concentration (1000, 5000, and 25000 units/ml) and the ratio of anticoagulant volume to blood volume in the syringe. Heparin is the most commonly used anticoagulant; an excess in the syringe causes a drop in $PaCO_2$. This problem seems to occur most frequently when blood is drawn from an indwelling arterial line. Such lines are routinely flushed with a heparin solution; failure to discard the first few cc's of aspirated blood will give excess heparin in the sample.

The pH change from excess anticoagulant is variable because heparin has a slightly acidic pH, offsetting any rise in blood pH when $PaCO_2$ falls. Because of all the variables, if too much heparin is used one can't reliably determine true blood gas values from the measured data. If the syringe is part of a commercial kit, follow the manufacturer's recommendations about how much anticoagulant to leave in the barrel. Otherwise, it is best to wet the inside of the syringe and needle with heparin and leave no visible accumulation before drawing blood.

4. SAMPLE CONTAINS AN AIR BUBBLE OR THE SAMPLE HAS BEEN LEFT OPEN TO AIR.

At sea level, the atmospheric PO_2 is about 160 mm Hg (.21 x 760 mm Hg). If the patient's PaO_2 is lower than 160 mm Hg and the sample contains an air bubble, or the syringe is left open to air, the PO_2 in the sample will rise. The degree of rise depends on the initial PaO_2 and how long the sample is exposed to air. Exposure of the sample to air is one possible explanation for a negative $P(A-a)O_2$. Conversely, if the patient's PaO_2 is higher than 160 mm Hg, the sample PO_2 will fall. Because room air contains almost no CO_2, the resulting $PaCO_2$ of any air-exposed sample can be expected to fall, and the resulting pH to rise.

Occasionally an air bubble enters the blood gas machine's intake tube and causes erroneous measurement. One result could be an apparent negative $P(A-a)O_2$. If a portion of the blood sample is also run independently in a co-oximeter, the problem can usually be diagnosed. For example, a patient breathing room air has a PaO_2 of 149 mm Hg, measured SaO_2 82%, normal %COHb and %MetHb. The reason for the falsely high PaO_2 is most likely an air bubble introduced into the machine tubing leading to the oxygen electrode.

5. SAMPLE NOT PLACED IN ICE.

Arterial blood samples should always be placed in a bag or container filled with ice before transport to the blood gas lab. Metabolizing blood cells alter blood gas values, principally PaO_2, quickly at normal body temperature (37°C), but much less so at 0°C (temperature of ice water). An iced sample should remain stable for at least an hour. Any sample not placed in ice should be tested within minutes after it is drawn, or otherwise discarded. The main effect of cellular metabolism is to decrease PO_2. Several studies have shown a remarkable fall in PaO_2 if the blood contains > 100,000 white blood cells/mm^3 ("leukocyte larceny"), even when the sample is on ice. A white cell count of this magnitude (usually in leukemics) should mandate special handling, i.e., running the sample immediately. Alternatively, check the patient's oxygen saturation by pulse oximetry, which is not affected by extreme leukocytosis (Sacchetti 1990).

6. INCORRECT FIO_2. Blood gases are usually reported with the FIO_2 entered on the report form. If the FIO_2 is incorrect, the blood gas data may make sense physiologically but be interpreted incorrectly. For example, if a patient is noted to be receiving "40% oxygen by face mask," but the mask was actually off the patient when the blood was drawn, oxygenation will seem worse than it actually is. Another example, fortunately less common, is when the patient is wearing the prescribed oxygen appliance, but the oxygen is disconnected or turned off at the source. Whenever PaO_2 is unexpectedly reduced in a patient receiving supplemental oxygen, the O_2 source should be checked.

7. CALCULATED SaO_2 INTERPRETED AS MEASURED SaO_2. This pitfall, extensively discussed in Chapter 5, is easy to avoid if you know how the blood gas lab reports SaO_2. Ideally, the lab should either *not* report a calculated SaO_2 or else note that the reported value represents a calculation and not an actual measurement. The person interpreting the data then has to realize that the calculated SaO_2 may be significantly higher than true (measured) SaO_2, in states of carbon monoxide intoxication and methemoglobinemia (see Chapter 5).

8. DATA PHYSIOLOGICALLY INCORRECT. This pitfall occurs when data violate normal human physiology, e.g., the data lead to a negative $P(A-a)O_2$ or a calculated bicarbonate value impossible to obtain from the measured $PaCO_2$ and pH. The origin of the former problem is usually an FIO_2 listed as "room air" when the patient is actually receiving supplemental oxygen (compare with Pitfall 6, which is the opposite problem). A physiologically-incorrect bicarbonate is usually traceable to a transcription error. For example, if a technician writes down "pH 7.42, $PaCO_2$ 38, HCO_3^- 34," you should immediately recognize a probable transcription error for HCO_3^- and not make any interpretation based on its spuriously high value.

9. **CONFUSION OVER EFFECT OF PATIENT'S TEMP-ERATURE.** Arterial blood is always analyzed at normal body temperature, 37°C, in the blood gas machine. If the patient is febrile, the measured PaO_2 and $PaCO_2$ will be *lower* than in the patient; gas molecules are slowed by the lower temperature of the machine and register less pressure. Conversely, if the patient is hypothermic, the measured PaO_2 and $PaCO_2$ will be *higher* than in the patient; gas molecules are speeded up by the higher temperature of the machine and register greater pressure. For each degree centigrade above or below 37°C, the change in PaO_2 is approximately 5 mm Hg and the change in $PaCO_2$ approximately 2 mm Hg. Thus a patient febrile to 39°, whose measured PaO_2 and $PaCO_2$ are 80 and 40 mm Hg, respectively, has a "true" or *in vivo* PaO_2 of 90 mm Hg, $PaCO_2$ of 44 mm Hg.

Some labs automatically correct for patient temperature, while others purposely do not. On balance, most physicians seem to feel that temperature correction is not necessary and that all blood gas data should be interpreted with reference to normal values at 37°C. It may also be true that a low PaO_2 in a hypothermic patient is just as adequate (because of decreased metabolism) as a normal PaO_2 in an afebrile patient.

In truth, we don't know what blood gas values "should be" when body temperature is abnormal. The pitfall is not in ignoring patient temperature for purposes of blood gas interpretation, but in making too much of the temperature correction. For most clinical purposes it is best not to bother with any correction. If data are already corrected don't 'convert back' but continue to interpret the data based on normal reference values.

Finally, it is important to make sure that sequential blood gases in a given patient are all handled the same way. If temperature correction is done to some arterial blood samples and not to others, a change in PaO_2, for example, may reflect only the correction and not any real change in the patient's condition.

10. **DATA REPORTED UNDER WRONG PATIENT'S NAME OR ID NUMBER.** This pitfall is easy to avoid if there are previous blood gas results and the current data are way out of line or they make no clinical sense (see Pitfall 12). The pitfall is

difficult to avoid if there are no previous blood gas data and the results seem to fit the wrong patient.

11. **VERBAL REPORT INCORRECT.** Sometimes people mis-remember blood gas data, then report incorrect information to someone else. A physician on a busy service might remember three sets of blood gas data but confuse which set goes with which patient. The incorrectly-reported data may make sense physiologically and even fit the clinical picture, but because the data belong to some other patient the wrong treatment is ordered. Anyone responsible for treatment based on blood gas data should make sure the data are accurate. This means not relying on verbal reports that are based on memory.

12. **DATA MAKE NO CLINICAL SENSE.** Although one cannot determine blood gas values clinically, sometimes data are clearly out of line for a given patient's clinical status. For example, a report of pH 7.21, $PaCO_2$ 23 mm Hg, should be suspect if the patient is alert, in no apparent respiratory distress and without any clinical disease to explain the data (e.g., not in a state of ketoacidosis). If data make no clinical sense the test should be repeated. The opposite pitfall may also be encountered (No. 13).

13. **CORRECT DATA ARE IGNORED.** This pitfall occurs when the data seem so abnormal for the patient that the physician assumes a lab or sampling error, but the data are in fact accurate. For example, PaO_2 *may* be very low even though the patient is not dyspneic at rest. In such cases one should not assume a lab or sampling error, but either repeat the blood gas test or measure the patient's SaO_2 with pulse oximetry. As with all lab tests, one must use experience and clinical judgment to decide which tests to believe, which to ignore, and which to repeat.

CHAPTER 10.

Quik-Course on Blood Gas Interpretation
(for Introduction, see Page xxi)

Four equations and three physiologic processes (Chapters 1 and 2)

Arterial blood gas data include both measured and derived values. To obtain the following information, an aliquot of arterial blood is entered into two different machines, a blood gas analyzer and a co-oximeter. HCO_3^-, base excess and arterial oxygen content (CaO_2) are calculations in most blood gas laboratories.

Normal Arterial Blood Gas Values*

pH	7.35-7.45
$PaCO_2$	35-45 mm Hg
PaO_2	> 70 mm Hg**
HCO_3^-	22-26 mEq/l
%MetHb	<1%
%COHb	<2.5%
Base excess	-2.0 to 2.0 mEq/L
CaO_2	16-22 ml O_2/dl

* At sea level, breathing ambient air
** age-dependent

Blood gas data provide useful information on three physiologic processes: alveolar ventilation, oxygenation and acid-base balance. Four equations aid in understanding these processes in the clinical setting:

Equation	Physiologic Process
1) $PaCO_2$ equation	Alveolar ventilation
2) Alveolar gas equation	Oxygenation
3) Oxygen content equation	Oxygenation
4) Henderson-Hasselbalch equation	Acid-base balance

PaCO$_2$ and alveolar ventilation (Chapter 3)

Alveolar ventilation is the amount of air, in L/min, that reaches the alveoli *and* takes part in gas exchange. Alveolar ventilation is the only process by which the body can excrete the huge amount of CO_2 produced by metabolism. The CO_2 enters tissue capillaries and travels to the lungs where it is excreted in the fresh air brought to the alveoli (the alveolar ventilation). In a steady state, the amount of CO_2 added to the blood equals the amount of CO_2 excreted by the lungs; in a typical resting individual, this is approximately 200 ml CO_2/min.

In a non-steady state PaCO$_2$ will go up if CO_2 production exceeds alveolar ventilation and will go down if alveolar ventilation exceeds CO_2 production. PaCO$_2$ is thus directly related to the rate of CO_2 production ($\dot{V}CO_2$) and inversely related to alveolar ventilation ($\dot{V}A$); this very important relationship is reflected in the PaCO$_2$ equation:

$$PaCO_2 = \frac{\dot{V}CO_2 \times .863}{\dot{V}A}$$

The constant ".863" converts different units for $\dot{V}CO_2$ (ml/min) and $\dot{V}A$ (L/min) into PaCO$_2$ units of mm Hg. Clinically, it is not necessary to know either $\dot{V}CO_2$ or $\dot{V}A$ but *only their ratio*, which is provided by PaCO$_2$. The following terms are used to characterize high, normal and low PaCO$_2$ values.

PaCO$_2$	Condition in blood	State of alveolar ventilation
> 45 mm Hg	Hypercapnia	Hypoventilation
35 - 45 mm Hg	Eucapnia	Normal ventilation
< 35 mm Hg	Hypocapnia	Hyperventilation

The terms hypo- and hyperventilation should be reserved for specific PaCO$_2$ measurements; they should not be used to characterize a patient's rate or depth of breathing, or degree of respiratory effort.

Hypercapnia is a common and serious respiratory problem. The PaCO$_2$ equation shows that the only physiologic reason for elevated PaCO$_2$ is inadequate alveolar ventilation for the amount of CO_2 production. Since alveolar ventilation ($\dot{V}A$) equals total ventilation ($\dot{V}E$) minus dead space ventilation ($\dot{V}D$), hypercapnia can arise from insufficient $\dot{V}E$, increased $\dot{V}D$, or a combination.

Examples of inadequate $\dot{V}E$:	sedative drug overdose
	respiratory muscle paralysis
	central hypoventilation
Examples of increased $\dot{V}D$:	chronic obstructive pulmonary disease
	severe restrictive lung disease (with
	shallow, rapid breathing)

The $PaCO_2$ equation shows why $PaCO_2$ cannot reliably be assessed clinically. Since you never know the patient's $\dot{V}CO_2$ or $\dot{V}A$, you cannot determine their ratio, which is what $PaCO_2$ provides.

There is no predictable correlation between $PaCO_2$ and the clinical picture. *Any combination of respiratory rate, depth, or effort can reflect any $PaCO_2$ value, and vice versa.* A patient in profound respiratory distress can have a high, normal, or low $PaCO_2$. A patient with no clinically apparent respiratory problem can have a high, normal, or low $PaCO_2$.

The bedside measurement of total or minute ventilation (tidal volume times respiratory rate) does not give the patient's $\dot{V}CO_2$ or $\dot{V}D$, and so does not provide any information about $\dot{V}A$ or $PaCO_2$. When there is concern about the adequacy of a patient's ventilation, $PaCO_2$ must be measured: invasively by arterial blood gas, or non-invasively by end-tidal PCO_2. Furthermore, once PCO_2 is measured it can only be interpreted in light of the full clinical picture.

Besides indicating a serious derangement in the respiratory system, hypercapnia poses a threat to the patient for three reasons:

- $PaCO_2$ inversely correlates with PAO_2 (equation 2)
- Increasing $PaCO_2$ leads to reduced pH (equation 4)
- The higher the baseline $PaCO_2$, the greater it will rise for any given fall in $\dot{V}A$ (e.g., a one L/min decrease in $\dot{V}A$ will raise the $PaCO_2$ a greater amount when the baseline is 50 mm Hg than when it is 40 mm Hg).

As stated previously, $PaCO_2$ is a component of formulas that help determine both oxygenation and acid-base status: the alveolar gas equation for alveolar PO_2 and the Henderson-Hasselbalch equation for pH. Both equations are discussed in the sections that follow.

■ ■ ■ ■ ■ ■ ■ ■ ■ ■ ■ ■ ■ ■ ■ ■

PaO$_2$, PAO$_2$ and the alveolar gas equation (Chapter 4)

PaO$_2$ is the partial pressure of oxygen in arterial blood, measured in mm Hg (units are sometimes called torr; 1 mm Hg = 1 torr). PaO$_2$ does not reveal how much oxygen is in the blood (see Oxygen Content), but only the pressure exerted by dissolved (unbound) O$_2$ molecules against the measuring electrode. PaO$_2$ is usually reduced in the presence of ventilation-perfusion (V-Q) imbalance, the physiologic state characteristic of all global airway and alveolar disease processes (e.g., asthma, atelectasis, bronchitis, pneumonia, pulmonary edema, pulmonary embolism).

The *upper* limit of PaO$_2$ is determined by the mean alveolar PO$_2$ (PAO$_2$). In a steady state, the measured PaO$_2$ should never be higher than the calculated PAO$_2$; a continuously "negative" A-a PO$_2$ difference is incompatible with life. The *lower* limit of PaO$_2$ is determined by several factors, mainly the extent of V-Q imbalance within the millions of alveolar-capillary units. Normal PaO$_2$ is age-dependent; breathing room air, at sea level, PaO$_2$ ranges from a high of 100 mm Hg in children down to the 70s in octogenarians: PaO$_2$ = 109 - .43(age in years). The normal decline of PaO$_2$ with age is due largely to natural loss of lung compliance, which causes a worsening of ventilation-perfusion imbalance.

Whereas PaO$_2$ is a laboratory measurement, PAO$_2$ is a calculation derived from the alveolar gas equation. In essence, PAO$_2$ equals the inspired PO$_2$ (PIO$_2$) minus the alveolar PCO$_2$ (PACO$_2$). Since PACO$_2$ is assumed equal to PaCO$_2$, the latter is used in the abbreviated form of this important equation:

$$PAO_2 = PIO_2 - 1.2 \,(PaCO_2)$$
where
$$PIO_2 = FIO_2 \,(P_B - 47).$$

PIO$_2$ is a function of the FIO$_2$ and barometric pressure; 47 mm Hg is the water vapor pressure at normal body temperature, and must be subtracted from P$_B$. Unlike PaO$_2$, PAO$_2$ is not age-dependent, but remains constant so long as the variables in the equation are unchanged.

Are the lungs transferring oxygen properly? The answer is found by the *difference* between calculated PAO$_2$ and measured PaO$_2$. This difference, P(A-a)O$_2$, is colloquially called the 'A-a gradient,' although it does not reflect a true gradient but rather a state of ventilation-perfusion imbalance within the lungs. The range for normal P(A-a)O$_2$ increases with age and FIO$_2$. When FIO$_2$ = 1.00, normal P(A-a)O$_2$ can range up to 110 mm Hg.

Without knowledge of PAO₂ one cannot properly interpret any PaO₂ value. Is a PaO_2 of 90 mm Hg normal? A PaO_2 of 28 mm Hg abnormal? You must know the variables in the alveolar gas equation to interpret properly any PaO_2 value. A PaO_2 of 90 mm Hg is normal in a subject with normal $PaCO_2$ breathing room air at sea level. The same PaO_2 would be abnormal in someone with a $PaCO_2$ of 25 mm Hg; the alveolar gas equation shows that the PAO_2 — and hence PaO_2 — should be higher by about 15 mm Hg, i.e., PAO_2 120 mm Hg, PaO_2 105 mm Hg. A PaO_2 of 90 mm Hg would also be abnormal — and indicate severely impaired lungs — in a patient breathing 100% oxygen at sea level. Under these conditions PAO_2 should be over 600 mm Hg with normal lungs, and PaO_2 at least 500 mm Hg.

In terms of oxygen transfer, a PaO_2 of 28 mm Hg would be normal on the summit of Mt. Everest (29,028 ft.) for a climber breathing pure mountain air. Barometric pressure at this altitude has been measured at only 253 mm Hg; with extreme hyperventilation (to 7.5 mm Hg), the resulting PAO_2 and PaO_2 were estimated at only 35 mm Hg and 28 mm Hg, respectively. A PaO_2 of 28 mm Hg would also be normal in someone inhaling only 8% oxygen. The subject in either situation is *hypoxemic*, but not because of any lung disease or defect in oxygen transfer.

In summary, PaO_2 must always be interpreted with knowledge of the $PaCO_2$, FIO_2 and barometric pressure, variables that are incorporated into the alveolar gas equation for PAO_2. A low PaO_2 with increased $P(A-a)O_2$ points to ventilation-perfusion imbalance and disease within the lungs. The vast majority of patients with low PaO_2 have ventilation-perfusion imbalance and so manifest an increased $P(A-a)O_2$. The following table lists this and other physiologic causes of a low PaO_2 and elevated $P(A-a)O_2$.

Causes of Low PaO₂	**P(A-a)O₂**
Non-respiratory	
Cardiac right to left shunt	Increased
Decreased PIO_2	Normal
Low mixed venous oxygen content	Increased
Respiratory	
Pulmonary right to left shunt	Increased
Ventilation-perfusion imbalance	Increased
Diffusion barrier	Increased
Hypoventilation (increased $PaCO_2$)	Normal

SaO₂ and oxygen content (Chapter 5)

Tissues need a requisite amount of oxygen molecules for metabolism. Neither the PaO_2 nor the SaO_2 tells *how much* oxygen is in the blood. *How much* is provided by the oxygen content, CaO_2 (units ml O_2/dl). CaO_2 is calculated as:

$$CaO_2 = \text{quantity } O_2 \text{ bound} + \text{quantity O2 dissolved}$$
$$\text{to hemoglobin} \qquad \text{in plasma}$$

$$CaO_2 = (Hb \times 1.34 \times SaO_2) + (.003 \times PaO_2).$$

The quantity of oxygen bound to hemoglobin is the product of the hemoglobin content (Hb, in gm/dl), the oxygen carrying capacity of hemoglobin (1.34 ml O_2/gm Hb), and the oxygen saturation of hemoglobin in arterial blood (SaO_2). The quantity of oxygen dissolved in plasma is the product of its solubility constant (.003 ml O_2/dl/mm Hg) and the PaO_2 in mm Hg.

Hypoxemia can be broadly defined as 'low oxygen' in the blood. Hypoxemia is more specifically characterized by a reduced PaO_2, SaO_2, *or* CaO_2. Hypoxia is a more general term than hypoxemia; it signifies reduced oxygen to the body as a whole, and includes all causes of hypoxemia.

Causes of Hypoxia - A General Classification

1. Hypoxemia
   a. reduced PaO_2 - most commonly from lung disease (physiologic mechanism: V-Q imbalance)
   b. reduced SaO_2 - most commonly from reduced PaO_2; other possible causes include carbon monoxide poisoning, methemoglobinemia, or rightward shift of the O_2-dissociation curve
   c. reduced hemoglobin content - anemia

2. Reduced oxygen delivery to the tissues
   a. reduced cardiac output - shock, congestive heart failure
   b. left to right systemic shunt (as may be seen in septic shock)

3. Decreased tissue oxygen uptake
   a. mitochondrial poisoning (e.g., cyanide poisoning)
   b. left-shifted hemoglobin dissociation curve (e.g., from acute alkalosis, excess CO, or abnormal hemoglobin structure)

CARBOXYHEMOGLOBIN. Every blood gas lab measures PaO_2 but not all measure SaO_2; some labs calculate SaO_2 based on the PaO_2 and a standard oxygen dissociation curve (adjusted for the patient's measured pH and temperature). A calculated SaO_2 is potentially hazardous as it will miss two important causes of hypoxemia that lower SaO_2 without affecting PaO_2: carbon monoxide poisoning and methemoglobinemia.

Carbon monoxide is a colorless, odorless gas that results from incomplete combustion of hydrocarbon fuels. It causes hypoxemia two ways. First, CO displaces O_2 from hemoglobin to form carboxyhemoglobin (COHb), and thereby reduces the SaO_2 and oxygen content. Second, CO shifts the oxygen dissociation curve *to the left*. As a result of the left shift, oxygen that is taken up by hemoglobin is held *more tightly than normal*, making less O_2 available to the tissues for any given PO_2 value.

Normal %COHb is less than 3% in urban dwellers. Between 5% and 10% COHb is commonly found in cigarette and cigar smokers. Symptoms begin at higher values, with coma and death occurring above 50% COHb. Excess COHb should always be suspected if the *measured* SaO_2 is significantly lower than predicted for the PaO_2 (e.g., PaO_2 80 mm Hg with a measured SaO_2 of 75%). The diagnosis is confirmed by direct measurement of %COHb. Modern co-oximeters can measure both SaO_2 and %COHb.

Note that pulse oximeters *do not* distinguish between oxyhemoglobin and carboxyhemoglobin and so cannot be used to detect carbon monoxide intoxication. A patient with 30% COHb and a true (if measured with a co-oximeter) SaO_2 of 65% will have a pulse oximeter SaO_2 reading of 95%.

METHEMOGLOBIN. Normal hemoglobin contains iron in the ferrous or Fe^{++} state. It is in this state that hemoglobin binds to oxygen in the pulmonary capillaries. Methemoglobin contains iron in the ferric or Fe^{+++} state, which makes the hemoglobin unable to bind oxygen. This 'oxidized' hemoglobin state is usually caused by a drug reaction (to nitrates, topical anesthetics, etc.) and is reversible with time (severe cases are treated with the reducing agent methylene blue). Like COHb, excess methemoglobin does not lower PaO_2 but only SaO_2. Methemoglobin can be directly measured by a co-oximeter, or suspected by the presence of intense cyanosis in a patient with normal PaO_2. Unlike CO, excess methemoglobin depresses the pulse oximeter reading of SaO_2 somewhat, but not linearly (see Chapter 5 for further discussion of this topic).

■ ■ ■ ■ ■ ■ ■ ■ ■ ■ ■ ■ ■ ■ ■ ■

pH and the Henderson-Hasselbalch equation (Chapter 6)

The concentration of hydrogen ion is related to the concentration of carbonic acid and bicarbonate. The Henderson-Hasselbalch equation defines the hydrogen ion concentration in terms of pH as follows:

$$pH = pK + \log \frac{[HCO_3^-]}{.03\,[PaCO_2]}$$

pH is a confusing term for acidity, since small numerical changes represent large and *opposite* changes in hydrogen ion concentration, $[H^+]$. A pH change of 1.00 represents a 10-fold change in $[H^+]$. Thus

pH	$[H^+]$ in nanomoles/L
7.00	100
7.30	50
7.40	40
7.50	32
8.00	10

Clinical and physiologic acid-base disorders do not always lead to predictable changes in the blood. Any given set of blood gases (e.g., low pH, low $PaCO_2$, low HCO_3^-) can come from several pathways and represent many different clinical disorders. By convention, terms ending in "emia" apply to blood changes only; terms ending in "osis" apply to physiologic processes which may or may not lead to particular changes in the blood. The following terminology is now widely accepted in describing and discussing acid base disorders.

Acidemia: blood pH < 7.35

Acidosis: a primary physiologic process that, occurring alone, tends to cause acidemia. Examples: metabolic acidosis from low-perfusion lactic acidosis; respiratory acidosis from acute hypoventilation. If the patient also has an alkalosis at the same time, the resulting blood pH may be low, normal or high.

Alkalemia: blood pH > 7.45

Alkalosis: a primary physiologic process that, occurring alone, tends to cause alkalemia. Examples: metabolic alkalosis from excessive diuretic therapy; respiratory alkalosis from acute hyperventilation. If the patient also has an acidosis at the same time, the resulting blood pH may be high, normal or low.

Primary acid-base disorder: One of the four acid-base disturbances that is manifested by an initial change in HCO_3^- or $PaCO_2$. If HCO_3^- changes first, the disorder is either a metabolic acidosis (reduced HCO_3^- and acidemia) or metabolic alkalosis (elevated HCO_3^- and alkalemia). If $PaCO_2$ changes first, the problem is either respiratory alkalosis (reduced $PaCO_2$ and alkalemia) or respiratory acidosis (elevated $PaCO_2$ and acidemia).

Compensation: The change in HCO_3^- or $PaCO_2$ that results from the primary event. Compensatory changes are not classified by the terms used for the four primary acid-base disturbances. For example, a patient who hyperventilates (lowers $PaCO_2$) solely as compensation for metabolic acidosis does *not* have a respiratory alkalosis. Since the hyperventilation occurs solely as compensation for metabolic acidosis there is no respiratory alkalosis, the latter being a primary disorder that, alone, would lead to alkalemia. In simple, uncomplicated metabolic acidosis the patient will never develop alkalemia.

Primary acid-base disorders

The four primary acid-base disorders are defined below; some clinical causes for each are listed on the next page.

Respiratory alkalosis - A primary disorder where the first change is a lowering of $PaCO_2$, resulting in an elevated pH. Compensation is a secondary lowering of bicarbonate by the kidneys; this reduction in HCO_3^- is not metabolic acidosis, since it is not a primary process.

Respiratory acidosis - A primary disorder where the first change is an elevation of $PaCO_2$, resulting in decreased pH. Compensation is a secondary retention of bicarbonate by the kidneys; this elevation of HCO_3^- is not metabolic alkalosis, since it is not a primary process.

Metabolic Acidosis - A primary acid-base disorder where the first change is a lowering of HCO_3^-, resulting in decreased pH. Compensation is a secondary hyperventilation by the respiratory system; this lowering of $PaCO_2$ is not respiratory alkalosis, since it is not a primary process. Metabolic acidosis is conveniently divided into elevated and normal anion gap acidosis. Anion gap, AG, is calculated as

$$AG = Na^+ - (Cl^- + CO_2).$$

The normal AG calculated in this manner is 12 +/- 4 mEq/L. (CO_2 in this equation is the "total CO_2" measured in the chemistry lab as part of routine serum electrolytes, and consists mostly of bicarbonate. If AG is calculated using K^+, the normal gap is 16 +/- 4 mEq/L.) High anion gap acidosis arises from excess acid added to the blood that has an unmeasured anion, e.g., lactic acidosis (lactate anion). Normal AG acidosis arises from excess acid added to the blood with the measured anion as chloride, or to loss of bicarbonate (see Table, below).

Metabolic alkalosis - A primary acid-base disorder where the first change is an elevation of HCO_3^-, resulting in increased pH. Metabolic alkalosis can occur from excess bicarbonate added to the blood, or from loss of HCl. The former can occur from administration of alkali or from excess renal reabsorption HCO_3^- (common with diuretic therapy). GI loss of HCl is common with nasogastric suctioning and vomiting. Compensation is a secondary hypoventilation; this raising of $PaCO_2$ is not respiratory acidosis, since it is not a primary process. Compensation for metabolic alkalosis is less predictable than for the other three acid-base disorders (see Chapter 6 for further discussion).

Some Clinical Causes of the Four Primary Acid-Base Disorders

Metabolic acidosis
with increased anion gap
lactic acidosis
ketoacidosis
with normal anion gap
diarrhea
some cases of renal insufficiency

Metabolic alkalosis
diuretics
corticosteroids
nasogastric suctioning or vomiting of gastric contents

Respiratory acidosis (= respiratory failure)
central nervous system depression (e.g., drug overdose)
chest bellows dysfunction (e.g., myasthenia gravis)
disease of lungs and/or upper airway (e.g., chronic obstructive lung disease, severe asthma attack, severe pulmonary edema)

Respiratory alkalosis
hypoxemia (includes altitude)
anxiety
sepsis
any acute pulmonary insult, e.g., pneumonia, mild asthma attack, mild pulmonary edema

Mixed Acid-Base Disorders

Often there is more than one acid-base disorder in the same patient at the same time. The following observations are useful in diagnosing mixed acid-base disorders:

1. Single acid-base disorders do not lead to normal blood pH. A truly normal pH with distinctly abnormal HCO_3^- or $PaCO_2$ indicates two or more primary disorders. Example: pH 7.40, $PaCO_2$ 20 mm Hg, HCO_3^- 12 mEq/L.

2. Plasma bicarbonate changes with acute changes in $PaCO_2$. Such changes in HCO_3^- are instantaneous and have *nothing* to do with renal compensation, which begins hours later. Extreme acute hyperventilation can lower HCO_3^- to about 15 mEq/L and extreme acute hypoventilation can raise it to about 29 mEq/L; a HCO_3^- outside this range must indicate either a renal compensatory mechanism or a primary metabolic acid-base disorder.

3. The biochemical changes with acute hyper- and hypoventilation point to another useful clue to the presence of a mixed acid-base disorder: a higher- or lower-than-expected bicarbonate value with *any* change in $PaCO_2$. Thus a slightly low HCO_3^- concentration in the presence of hypercapnia suggests a concomitant metabolic acidosis (e.g., $PaCO_2$ 50 mm Hg, pH 7.27, HCO_3^- 22 mEq/L); a slightly elevated HCO_3^- in the presence of hypocapnia suggests a concomitant metabolic alkalosis (e.g., $PaCO_2$ 30 mm Hg, pH 7.56, HCO_3^- 26 mEq/L).

4. Acute respiratory disorders can be expressed by regression equations that predict pH or HCO_3^- for a given change in $PaCO_2$. Useful approximations of these equations include the following statements.

    a) in <u>acute respiratory acidosis</u> up to $PaCO_2$ of 70 mm Hg,
        for every 10 mm Hg ↑ in $PaCO_2$:
        pH ↓ by ~ 0.07 units and HCO_3^- ↑ by ~ 1 mEq/L.

    b) in <u>acute respiratory alkalosis</u> down to $PaCO_2$ 20 mm Hg,
        for every 10 mm Hg ↓ in $PaCO_2$:
        pH ↑ by ~ 0.08 units and HCO_3^- ↓ by ~ 2 mEq/L.

    c) in fully compensated <u>metabolic acidosis</u>, the numerical value of $PaCO_2$ should be the same (or close to) the last two digits of arterial pH, e.g., pH 7.25, $PaCO_2$ 25 mm Hg.

In summary, steps to proper acid-base diagnosis and management include:

- Determine that the patient has an acid-base disorder from arterial blood gas and/or serum electrolyte measurements.

- Use a full clinical assessment (history, physical examination, other laboratory data) to explain the disorder in terms of physiologic processes and underlying clinical condition(s).

- Aim toward correcting the pH, particularly if it is outside the range of 7.30 - 7.52 ($[H^+]$ = 50 to 30 nMole/L); the danger to the patient is not the absolute value of HCO_3^- or $PaCO_2$, but the abnormal pH.

- Treat the underlying clinical condition.

APPENDIX A: POST-TEST

If you achieve over 90% correct responses on the Post-test, chances are you have learned all you really need to know about arterial blood gas interpretation. Congratulations!

<u>Directions</u>: For each of the following seven statements or questions there may be none, one, or more than one correct response. Circle the correct response(s) *before* checking your answers.

1. Carbon monoxide
   a) shifts the O_2-dissociation curve to the left.
   b) lowers the PaO_2.
   c) increases the P_{50}.
   d) lowers the CaO_2.
   e) poisoning is treated with a high FIO_2.

2. A patient with $PaCO_2$ 75 mm Hg and HCO_3^- 23 mEq/L most likely has
   a) acute respiratory acidosis as an isolated primary acid-base disorder.
   b) respiratory acidosis plus metabolic acidosis.
   c) a $PaO_2 < 70$ mm Hg if the blood gas was obtained while the patient was breathing room air.
   d) a low arterial pH.
   e) a low serum sodium.

3. Pulse oximetry is generally not accurate in patients
   a) with carbon monoxide intoxication.
   b) with poor perfusion of extremities.
   c) of African-American descent.
   d) who are acutely hyperventilating.
   e) who are receiving supplemental oxygen.

(continued)

(continued)

4. Which of the following statements about hemoglobin
    is/are correct?
    a) Oxidized hemoglobin contains iron in the 3^+ or
       oxidized state and cannot bind oxygen.
    b) De-oxygenated hemoglobin contains iron in the 2^+
       or ferrous state and is unbound to oxygen.
    c) Oxygenated hemoglobin contains iron in the 2^+ or
       ferrous state and is bound to oxygen.
    d) Carboxyhemoglobin contains iron in the 2^+ or
       ferrous state but not in the 3^+ or ferric state.
    e) An SaO_2 of 95% means that 95% of the heme
       binding sites are bound with oxygen.

5. A 49-year-old alcoholic is admitted to hospital after
    three days of vomiting. Arterial blood gas and
    electrolyte values (on room air):

pH	7.50	Na^+	130 mEq/L
$PaCO_2$	53 mm Hg	K^+	2.3 mEq/L
PaO_2	55 mm Hg	CO_2	24 mEq/L
SaO_2	88%	Cl^-	76 mEq/L

    Which of the following disorder(s) is(are) likely
    present?
    a) metabolic acidosis
    b) metabolic alkalosis
    c) respiratory alkalosis
    d) respiratory acidosis
    e) ventilation-perfusion imbalance

(continued)

(continued)

6.   A 65 year-old patient with severe emphysema is sitting
     in bed, breathing room air at a respiratory rate of
     23/minute. Arterial blood gas values at this time show:

     pH   7.35
     $PaCO_2$ 65 mm Hg
     PaO_2 45 mm Hg
     SaO_2 78%
     hemoglobin content   10 gm%

     Which of the following problems reasonably explain(s)
     the reduced oxygen content?

     a)   ventilation-perfusion imbalance
     b)   anemia
     c)   excess carbon monoxide
     d)   hypercapnia
     e)   left shift of the oxygen dissociation curve

7.   In the clinical setting, which of the following are valid
     statements concerning blood gas physiology?
     a)   End-tidal PCO_2 should always be higher than
          arterial PCO_2.
     b)   Alveolar PO_2 should always be higher than arterial
          PO_2.
     c)   The %oxyhemoglobin + %carboxyhemoglobin +
          %methemoglobin should never exceed 100%.
     d)   The ratio of dead space to tidal volume should
          never exceed 1.0.
     e)   The average airway pressure does not exceed
          barometric pressure in a spontaneously breathing
          patient.

END OF POST-TEST

APPENDIX B: ANSWERS

Answers to Pre-test questions

1. a and b are correct
   incorrect:
   c) patient may have other reasons to hyperventilate, such as asthma exacerbation, fever, any acute parenchymal infiltrate
   d) patient may be breathing deeper than normal
   e) patient could have metabolic acidosis

2. b, c and e are correct
   incorrect:
   a) anemia reduces oxygen content, not PaO_2
   d) carbon monoxide reduces SaO_2 and CaO_2, not PaO_2

3. a and d are correct
   incorrect:
   b, c, and e; you need at least two of the three variables in the Henderson-Hasselbalch equation to obtain a reasonable idea of a patient's acid-base balance

4. a, b, c and d are correct
   incorrect:
   e) In theory, the bicarbonate calculated in the blood gas lab should be 1 to 2 mEq/L less than the "CO_2" calculated in the chemistry lab, since the latter value includes the quantity contributed by $PaCO_2$

5. c, d and e are correct
   incorrect:
   a) each *gram* of hemoglobin can combine with 1.34 ml of oxygen
   b) Normal CaO_2 is between 16 and 22 *ml O_2/dl*

Answers to Pre-test questions (continued)

6. a, c and e are correct
    incorrect:
    b) arterial PO_2 and pH are not directly related by any equation
    d) arterial PO_2 is related to SaO_2 by the O_2 dissociation curve, which has a sigmoid configuration

7. b and d are correct
    incorrect:
    a) "hyperventilation" and "hypoventilation" should only be used clinically as they relate to the $PaCO_2$
    c) people with normal lungs can increase arterial PO_2 above 100 mm Hg with hyperventilation
    e) a patient can have profound acid-base imbalance yet normal pH from opposing acid-base disorders (e.g., combined metabolic acidosis and metabolic alkalosis)

Answers to Post-test Questions

1. a, d and e are correct
    incorrect:
    b) PaO_2 is not affected
    c) the P_{50} is lower with a left-shifted curve

2. b, c and d are correct
    incorrect:
    a) the slightly lowered bicarbonate points to a metabolic acidosis
    e) there is no predictable correlation between serum

sodium and acid-base state

Answers to Post-test questions (continued)

3. a and b are correct
   incorrect:
   c-e) skin color, acute hyperventilation, and
   supplemental oxygen should not affect SaO_2 readings
   with modern pulse oximeters

4. all are correct

5. a, b, d and e are likely present
   incorrect:
   c) the patient is hypoventilating, not hyperventilating,
   as would be the case with respiratory alkalosis

6. a, b and d are correct
   incorrect:
   c) the SaO_2 of 88% is appropriate for a PaO_2 of 45
   mm Hg and this pH; these values do not suggest the
   presence of excess carbon monoxide
   e) with a low pH the oxygen dissociation curve would
   be shifted to the right

7. b, c, d and e are correct
   incorrect:
   a) end-tidal PCO_2 should always be *lower* than the
   arterial PCO_2

APPENDIX C: SYMBOLS AND ABBREVIATIONS

A	= alveolar
a	= arterial
AG	= anion gap
ABG	= arterial blood gas
BB	= buffer base
BE	= base excess
BUN	= blood urea nitrogen, an index of renal function
CaO_2	= content of oxygen in arterial blood, ml O_2/dl
Cl^-	= chloride
CO	= carbon monoxide
CO_2	= carbon dioxide; CO_2 is symbol for both CO_2 as a blood gas (measured as $PaCO_2$ in the ABG test, units mm Hg), and for the quantity of non-protein-bound CO_2 (measured with serum electrolytes, units mEq/L)
COHb	= carboxyhemoglobin, usually expressed as a percentage of the total hemoglobin, e.g. 10%, COHb
dl	= deciliter, 100 ml
DPG	= diphosphoglycerate
Fe	= iron
FEV-1	= forced expiratory volume in first second
FIO_2	= fraction of inspired oxygen, expressed either as a decimal (e.g., .21, 1.00) or a percentage (21%, 100%)
FVC	= forced vital capacity
gm	= gram
$[H^+]$	= hydrogen ion concentration, nanomoles/L
Hb	= hemoglobin
HCl	= hydrochloric acid
HCO_3^-	= bicarbonate
H-H	= Henderson-Hasselbalch
K^+	= potassium
L	= liter, 1000 ml
mEq/L	= milliequivalents/liter
metHb	= methemoglobin
min	= minute
ml	= milliliter

SYMBOLS AND ABBREVIATIONS (continued)

mm Hg = millimeters of mercury, standard unit for pressure; some texts use the term *torr*; 1 torr = 1 mm Hg

N_2 = nitrogen

Na^+ = sodium

O_2 = oxygen

P or p = pressure

P_{50} = PaO_2 at which 50% of the hemoglobin binding sites are combined with oxygen

$P(A\text{-}a)O_2$ = difference between calculated alveolar PO_2 and measured arterial PO_2

P_B = barometric pressure

$PetCO_2$ = partial pressure of CO_2 measured on an end-tidal sample of expired air

pH = symbol for negative logarithm of the hydrogen ion concentration, nanomoles/L

P_{H20} = water vapor pressure

PIO_2 = pressure of inspired oxygen

pK = negative logarithm of the dissociation constant for carbonic acid

R = respiratory quotient

SaO_2 = saturation of hemoglobin with oxygen in arterial blood

torr = unit of pressure; 1 torr = 1 mm Hg

V = a volume, e.g., VD = volume of dead space, ml or L

$\dot{V}$ = volume per unit time, e.g., $\dot{V}A$ = alveolar ventilation in L/min

VA = alveolar volume, ml or L

VD = dead space volume, ml or L

V/Q = ventilation/perfusion or ventilation-perfusion; some texts place a dot above each value, omitted here

VT = tidal volume, ml or L

$\dot{V}A$ = alveolar ventilation, L/min

$\dot{V}D$ = dead space ventilation, L/min

$\dot{V}E$ = minute ventilation, L/min (usually measured on an expired sample, hence the E)

APPENDIX D: GLOSSARY

acetazolamide - a carbonic anhydrase inhibitor that prevents reabsorption of HCO_3^- in the renal tubule. Used as a drug in some cases of metabolic alkalosis to lower serum HCO_3^-; also used to prevent high-altitude sickness.

acidemia - acid in blood; term used when arterial pH < 7.35.

acidosis - a physiologic process that, occurring alone, leads to an acidemia. Clinical causes include low-perfusion lactic acidosis (metabolic acidosis) and hypoventilation (respiratory acidosis).

air - the mixture of gases that makes up earth's atmosphere; contains 78% nitrogen, 21% oxygen, 1% other gases.

alkalemia - alkali in blood; term used when arterial pH > 7.45.

alkalosis - a physiologic process that, occurring alone, leads to an alkalemia. Causes include diuretic therapy (metabolic alkalosis) and acute hyperventilation (respiratory alkalosis).

alveolar-arterial PO_2 difference - difference between calculated mean alveolar PO_2 and measured arterial PO_2; colloquially called 'A-a gradient' and annotated $P(A-a)O_2$. Elevation of $P(A-a)O_2$ usually signifies ventilation-perfusion imbalance within the lungs.

alveolar gas equation - equation for calculating PAO_2, the mean alveolar PO_2: $PAO_2 = PIO_2 - 1.2(PaCO_2)$.

alveolar ventilation - $\dot{V}A$; the volume of air per minute that enters alveoli and takes part in gas exchange; is equal to total (minute) ventilation minus dead space ventilation.

anion gap - the difference between the serum sodium, and the sum of chloride and bicarbonate, concentrations; normal AG is 12 +/- 4 mEq/L. An elevated AG signifies excess unmeasured anions and a state of metabolic acidosis.

atmosphere - the gaseous blanket between the surface of the earth and outer space, approximate 150 miles depth.

barometric pressure - P_B; pressure of the atmosphere at a given altitude. At sea level average P_B is 760 mm Hg, i.e., it will support a closed column of mercury 760 mm high.

base excess - difference between the normal quantity of total buffer base ([BB]) and the [BB] calculated on a blood sample. Normal BE is 0 +/- 2 mEq/L. An increase in BE correlates with an increase in serum bicarbonate; a decreased in BE (negative BE) correlates with reduced bicarbonate.

bicarbonate - HCO_3^-; one of two buffer components of the bicarbonate buffering system; normal value is 24 +/- 2 mEq/L.

blood gas - any gas dissolved in blood, e.g., oxygen, nitrogen, carbon dioxide, carbon monoxide, etc; also refers generically to test that measures partial pressure of oxygen (PO_2) and carbon dioxide (PCO_2), and pH.

bronchitis - inflammation of the airways; may be acute or chronic. Chronic bronchitis is often associated with cigarette smoking and may lead to chronic obstructive pulmonary disease.

carbon dioxide - CO_2; gaseous byproduct of animal metabolism and major determinant of acidity of blood. Partial pressure of CO_2 is routinely measured as part of arterial blood gases.

carbon monoxide - CO; colorless, odorless gas that combines avidly with hemoglobin to form carboxyhemoglobin; small amounts of inhaled CO can cause profound hypoxemia. Symptoms of CO poisoning usually begin when level of carboxyhemoglobin exceeds 10%.

carboxyhemoglobin - hemoglobin bound with carbon monoxide.

chronic obstructive pulmonary disease - COPD; disease manifested by obstruction of the larger airways (> 2 mm diameter) that does not normalize despite optimal therapy. COPD can be divided into two broad diseases, chronic bronchitis and emphysema, both conditions usually caused by long term cigarette smoking.

compensation - alteration of HCO_3^- or $PaCO_2$ in direct response to a primary acid-base disturbance, e.g., hyperventilation as a compensation for metabolic acidosis.

confidence band - area on an acid-base map that includes 95% of the compensatory responses of a group of subjects to one of the four primary acid-base disorders.

co-oximeter - machine capable of measuring SaO_2, carboxyhemoglobin, methemoglobin and hemoglobin content on a single blood sample. Co-oximeter is used in blood gas labs in addition to the blood gas analyzer, which measures PO_2, PCO_2 and pH.

cyanosis - blue color in skin and mucous membranes usually apparent when desaturated (reduced) hemoglobin content in capillaries exceeds 5 gm/dl.

dead space - space that contains air but doesn't allow for gas exchange. 'Anatomic dead space' is made up of all non-alveolar air spaces (upper airway and all bronchi including terminal bronchioles). 'Physiologic dead space' includes all anatomic dead space plus those alveolar spaces that don't take part in gas exchange. Anatomic dead space is fixed in a given patient. Physiologic dead space varies according to the extent and severity of ventilation-perfusion imbalance.

dead space ventilation - the volume of air per minute that enters the airways (including alveoli) and does not take part in gas exchange; the volume of air that enters the physiologic dead space each minute. Dead space ventilation equals total (minute) ventilation minus alveolar ventilation.

denitrogenation - process of removing nitrogen from blood by inhaling 100% oxygen.

diffusion - physiologic process by which respiratory gases are exchanged across cell membranes; all diffusion in the respiratory system takes place from a region of higher gas pressure across a permeable membrane to a region of lower gas pressure.

electrolytes - positively or negatively charged ions in the blood; the most commonly measured electrolytes include sodium (Na^+), potassium (K^+), bicarbonate (HCO_3^-) and chloride (Cl^-).

emphysema - one type of chronic obstructive pulmonary disease; manifested by destruction of alveolar-capillary membranes and increased ventilation-perfusion imbalance.

end-capillary - in the pulmonary circulation, the last section of capillary that exchanges gases with the alveoli; in normal lungs the end-capillary PO_2 and PCO_2 of an individual gas exchange unit are assumed to equal the corresponding alveolar PO_2 and PCO_2, respectively.

end-tidal - the last portion of exhaled tidal volume; in normal lungs the end-tidal PCO_2 is assumed equal to the alveolar PCO_2, since alveolar gas is the last portion to leave the lungs during exhalation.

ferric - iron in the oxidized state, Fe^{+++}; heme groups that contain ferric iron cannot bind oxygen.

ferrous - iron in its normal state combined with hemoglobin, Fe^{++}.

FEV-1 - forced expiratory volume in first second; that portion of the forced vital capacity exhaled in first second of effort.

flow - volume per unit time, e.g., L/min, L/sec.

forced vital capacity - FVC; volume of air that can be rapidly and forcibly exhaled after a maximal inhalation.

gas - any matter that will expand in three dimensions to fill the available space.

helium - a lightweight, inert gas; used to measure lung volumes in the helium-dilution lung function test.

heme - iron-porphyrin portion of hemoglobin that chemically binds with oxygen.

hemoglobin - iron-porphyrin-protein complex that chemically binds oxygen, thus allowing for much greater oxygen carrying capacity than can be achieved from dissolved oxygen alone. Each molecule of hemoglobin is capable of combining with four molecules of oxygen.

Henderson-Hasselbalch equation - equation for calculating pH when the HCO_3^- and $PaCO_2$ are known.

hypercapnia - elevated $PaCO_2$ (> 45 mm Hg).

hypercarbia - elevated HCO_3^-; calculated plasma HCO_3^- > 26 mEq/L.

hyperventilation - excessive alveolar ventilation for the amount of CO_2 production; hyperventilation results in a fall in $PaCO_2$.

hypocapnia - reduced $PaCO_2$ (< 35 mm Hg).

hypocarbia - reduced HCO_3^-; calculated plasma HCO_3^- < 22 mEq/L.

hypoventilation - alveolar ventilation decreased for the amount of CO_2 production; hypoventilation results in a rise in $PaCO_2$.

hypoxemia - reduced PaO_2 and/or arterial oxygen content, e.g., PaO_2 < 60 mm Hg or SaO_2 < 90%.

hypoxia - general reduction in oxygen delivery, either because of hypoxemia, decreased cardiac output or decreased oxygen uptake in the systemic capillaries.

inert gas - a gas that does not enter into any chemical reaction with another substance; examples include hydrogen, helium, nitrogen, argon.

metabolic acidosis - a primary physiologic process that, occurring alone, causes acidemia by lowering HCO_3^-. Causes include low-perfusion lactic acidosis, keto-acidosis, aspirin overdose.

metabolic alkalosis - a primary physiologic process that, occurring alone, causes alkalemia by raising HCO_3^-. Causes include diuretic therapy, corticosteroids, nasogastric suction.

methemoglobin - hemoglobin that contains iron in its oxidized state, Fe^{+++}; in this state hemoglobin cannot bind oxygen.

minute ventilation - same as total ventilation; the amount of air inhaled or exhaled per minute. By convention, minute ventilation is measured on exhalation and is symbolized $\dot{V}$ E.

mixed venous - blood in the pulmonary artery, i.e., blood that is a mixture of the total venous return to the right side of the heart.

nanomole - one billionth of a mole; hydrogen ions are quantified in nanomoles, e.g., a pH of 7.40 represents a $[H^+]$ of 40 nanomoles/L.

nitrogen - inert gas that makes up 78% of air.

reduced hemoglobin - hemoglobin that is not combined with oxygen; contains iron in its normal, ferrous state (Fe^{++}).

obstructive impairment - term for decreased air flow through the bronchi; usually manifested by reduction in ratio of FEV-1 second to forced vital capacity.

oxidized hemoglobin - hemoglobin that contains iron in its oxidized state, Fe^{+++}; synonymous with methemoglobin.

oximetry - non-invasive method of measuring arterial oxygen saturation; modern machines measure pulse at the same time, hence test is sometimes referred to as 'pulse oximetry.'

oxygen - respirable gas essential to life; oxygen makes up 21% of the atmosphere.

oxygen content - the quantity of oxygen in the blood, expressed as ml O_2/dl.

oxygen dissociation curve - sigmoid curve obtained when values for

SaO_2 are plotted in relation to corresponding PaO_2 values. Shifts of the O_2-dissociation curve to the right or to the left can affect oxygen delivery to the tissues.

oxygen saturation - the percentage of total hemoglobin binding sites chemically combined with oxygen; maximum is 100%. Normal oxygen saturation is 95-98%.

partial pressure - pressure exerted by a single gas; partial pressure is unaffected by any other gases that may be present. The sum of all partial pressures equals the total gas pressure, which in air is the same as barometric pressure.

peak flow - maximal flow rate (in L/min or L/sec) attained on forced exhalation after maximal inhalation.

perfusion - amount of blood circulating to an area or organ, per minute.

physiologic dead space - volume of all airways, including alveoli, that contain air but do not participate in gas exchange.

pressure - force exerted by molecules; gas pressure is determined by number and speed of molecules that make up the gas. All gases exert pressure when free and uncombined chemically with a non-gas molecule. When oxygen or carbon dioxide chemically combine with hemoglobin, they no longer exert any pressure.

respiratory acidosis - acid-base state manifested by elevated $PaCO_2$ and reduced pH.

respiratory alkalosis - acid-base state manifested by reduced $PaCO_2$ and elevated pH.

respiratory failure - any state manifested by a low PaO_2 and/or high $PaCO_2$ when due to a defect in the respiratory system; term is usually applied when PaO_2 is less than 60 mm Hg or $PaCO_2$ > 50 mm Hg while breathing room air at sea level; different criteria apply for other conditions.

restrictive impairment - respiratory impairment manifested by inability to inhale maximally; may be caused by space occupying lesions in the lungs, pulmonary fibrosis, neuromuscular weakness, obesity, etc.

shunt - the term used for blood flowing through the lungs that does not come into contact with air; a shunt may be from anatomic causes (e.g., an arterio-venous fistula) or physiologic causes. Physiologic shunt occurs when alveoli become unventilated (e.g., from atelectasis) but remain perfused (V-Q of zero for those units).

spirometry - breathing test that measures vital capacity and its subdivisions.

supplemental oxygen - any amount of oxygen delivered to a patient greater than in the atmosphere; in clinical medicine, any $FIO_2 > 21\%$.

tidal volume - volume inhaled or exhaled during a normal quiet breath.

torr - unit of pressure; one torr = one mm Hg.

ventilation - amount of air entering the lungs per minute; the total or minute ventilation is the sum of dead space and alveolar ventilation.

ventilation-perfusion - also written as "ventilation/perfusion"; the ratio of ventilation to perfusion in a single alveolus, a region of the lungs, or both lungs.

ventilation-perfusion imbalance - the situation when there is more, or less, ventilation for the amount of perfusion to an alveolus or a group of alveoli. Ventilation-perfusion imbalance is the main physiologic cause of a decrease in PaO_2; this comes about when some lung units are relatively under-ventilated or relatively over-perfused. Many lung diseases lead to a state of ventilation-perfusion imbalance.

APPENDIX E: BIBLIOGRAPHY

References quoted in text — listed in alphabetical order

Arbus GS, Hebert LA, Levesque PR, et al. Characterization and clinical application of the "significance band" for acute respiratory alkalosis. N Engl J Med 1969;280:117-23.

Asch MJ, Dell RB, Williams GS, Cohen M, Winters RW. Time course for development of respiratory compensation in metabolic acidosis. J Lab Clin Med 1969;73:610-15.

Barker SJ, Tremper KK. The effect of carbon monoxide inhalation on pulse oximetry and transcutaneous PO_2. Anesthesiology 1987;66:677-79.

Barker SJ, Tremper KK, Hyatt J. Effects of methemoglobin-emia on pulse oximetry and mixed venous oximetry. Anesthesiology 1989;70:112-17.

Brackett NC Jr, Cohen JJ, Schwartz WB. Carbon dioxide titration curve of normal man. N Engl J Med 1965;272:6-12.

Cinel D, Markwell K, Lee R, Szidon P. Variability of the respiratory gas exchange ratio during arterial puncture. Am Rev Respir Dis 1991;143:217-18.

Clark LC Jr. Monitoring and control of blood and tissue O_2 tensions. Trans Am Soc Artif Intern Organs 1956;2:41.

Clark LC Jr, Wolf R, Granger D, Taylor Z. Continuous recording of blood oxygen tensions by polarography. J Appl Physiol 1953;6:189.

Comroe JH Jr. *Physiology of Respiration*, 2nd ed. Mosby-Year Book, Chicago, 1974.

Comroe JH Jr, Botelho S. The unreliability of cyanosis in the recognition of arterial hypoxemia. Am J Med Sci 1947; 214:1.

Eisenkraft JB. Pulse oximeter desaturation due to methemoglobinemia. Anesthesiology 1988;68:279-82.

Gabow PA (principal discussant). Disorders associated with an altered anion gap. Kidney Int 1985;27:472-83.

Gabow PA, Kaehny WD, Fennessy PV, et al. Diagnostic importance of an increased serum anion gap. N Engl J Med 1980;303:854-58.

Goldberg M, Green S, Moss ML, et al. Computer-based instruction and diagnosis of acid-base disorders. JAMA 973; 223:269-75.

Harris EA, Kenyon AM, Nisbet HD, et al. The normal alveolar-arterial oxygen tension gradient in man. Clin Sci Mol Med 1974;46:89-104.

Hood I, Campbell EJM. Is pK OK? (editorial). N Engl J Med 1982;306:864.

Javaheri S. Compensatory hypoventilation in metabolic alkalosis. Chest 1982;81:296-301.

Javaheri S, Kazemi H. Metabolic alkalosis and hypoventilation in humans. Am Rev Respir Dis 1987:136;1011-16.

Lundsgaard C, Van Slyke DD. Cyanosis. Medicine 1923;2:1-76.

Martin L. Abbreviating the alveolar gas equation. An argument for simplicity. Respir Care 1986;31:40-44.

Martin L. *Pulmonary Physiology in Clinical Practice.* Mosby-Year Book, St. Louis, 1987.

Martin L, Khalil H. How much reduced hemoglobin is necessary to generate central cyanosis? Chest 1990;97:182-85.

Narins RG, Emmett M. Simple and mixed acid-base disorders: A practical approach. Medicine (Baltimore) 1980;59:161-87.

Oster JR, Perez GO, Materson BJ. Use of the anion gap in clinical medicine. South Med J 1988;81:229-37.

Pierce NF, Fedson DS, Brigham KL, Mitra RC, et al. The ventilatory response to acute acid-base deficit in humans. Ann Intern Med 1970;72:633-40.

Raemer DN, Elliott WR, Topulos G, et al. The theoretical effect of carboxyhemoglobin on the pulse oximeter. J Clin Monit 1989;5:246-49.

Ralston AC, Webb RK, Runciman WB. Potential errors in pulse oximetry. III: Effects of interference, dyes, dyshaemoglobins and other pigments. Anaesthesia 1991;46:291-95.

Sacchetti A, Grynn J, Pope A, Vasso S. Leukocyte larceny: spurious hypoxemia confirmed with pulse oximetry. J Emerg Med 1990;8:567-69.

Severinghaus JW. AHA! Chapter XVIII, in Astrup P, Severinghaus JW: *The History of Blood Gases, Acids and Bases*. Radiometer A/S, Copenhagen, 1986.

Sorbini CA, Grassi V, Solinas E, Muiesan G. Arterial oxygen tension in relation to age in healthy subjects. Respiration 1968;25:3-13.

Stadie WC. The oxygen of the arterial and venous blood in pneumonia and its relation to cyanosis. J Exp Med 1919; 30:215.

Watcha MF, Connor MT, Hing AV. Pulse oximetry in methemoglobinemia. Am J Dis Child 1989;143:845-47.

West JB, Hackett PH, Maret KH, et al. Pulmonary gas exchange on the summit of Mt. Everest, J Appl Physiol 1983;55:678-87.

Winters RW. Terminology of acid-base disorders. Ann Intern Med 1965;63:873-84.

Additional references recommended on the subject of blood gas
measurement and interpretation, and basic pulmonary physiology

Astrup P, Severinghaus JW. *The History of Blood Gases, Acids
and Bases.* Radiometer A/S, Copenhagen, 1986. Distributed
in U.S. by Butterworth-Heinemann, Stoneham, MA.

Berne RM, Levy MN. *Physiology,* 2nd ed. Mosby-Year Book, St.
Louis, 1988.

Burton GG, Hodgkin JE, Ward JJ. *Respiratory Care. A Guide
to Clinical Practice,* 3rd ed. J.B. Lippincott Co., Philadelphia,
1991.

Clark JS, Votteri B, Ariagno RI, et al. Noninvasive assessment of
blood gases: State of the art. Am Rev Respir Dis 1992;145:
220-232.

Clark LC Jr. Measurement of oxygen tension: A historical
perspective. Crit Care Med 1981;9:690-2.

Crystal RG, West JB, eds. *The Lung: Scientific Foundations.*
Chapter 5.3, "Pulmonary Gas Exchange," Vol II. Raven
Press, New York, 1991.

Filley GF. *Acid-Base and Blood Gas Regulation.* Lea & Febiger,
Philadelphia, 1971.

Guyton, AC. *Textbook of Medical Physiology,* 8th ed. W.B.
Saunders Co., Philadelphia, 1991.

Forster RE, DuBois AB, Briscoe WA, et al. *The Lung:
Physiologic Basis of Pulmonary Function Tests,* 3rd ed. Mosby-
Year Book, Chicago, 1986.

Jones NL. *Blood Gases and Acid-base Physiology,* 2nd ed.
Thieme Medical Publishers, New York, 1987.

Lane EE, Walker JF. *Clinical Arterial Blood Gas Analysis.*
Mosby-Year Book, Chicago, 1987.

Malley WJ. *Clinical Blood Gases. Application and Non-invasive
Alternatives.* W.B. Saunders Co., Philadelphia, 1990.

McCurdy DK. Mixed metabolic and respiratory acid-base disturbances: diagnosis and treatment. Chest 1972;62:35S-44S.

Murray JF. *The Normal Lung*, 2nd ed. W.B. Saunders Co., Philadelphia, 1986.

Ruppel GL. *Manual of Pulmonary Function Testing*, 5th ed. Mosby-Year Book, St. Louis, 1991.

Schwartz WB, Relman AS. A critique of the parameters used in evaluation of acid-base disorders. N Engl J Med 1963; 268:1382-88.

Shapiro BA, Harrison RA, Cane RD, and Kozlowski-Templin RL. *Clinical Application of Blood Gases*, 4th ed. Mosby-Year Book, Chicago, 1988.

Statement on acid-base terminology. Report of the ad hoc committee of the New York Academy of Sciences Conference, November 23-24, 1964. Ann Intern Med 1965; 63:885-90

Tisi GM. *Pulmonary Physiology in Clinical Medicine*, 3rd ed. Williams & Wilkins, Baltimore, 1992.

West JB. State of the art. Ventilation-perfusion relationships. Am Rev Respir Dis 1977;116:919-43.

West JB. *Respiratory Physiology — The Essentials*, 3rd ed. Williams & Wilkins, Baltimore, 1989.

West JB. *Pulmonary Pathophysiology — The Essentials*, 4th ed. Williams & Wilkins, Baltimore, 1991.

West JB. *Ventilation/Blood Flow and Gas Exchange*, 5th ed. Oxford: Blackwell Scientific Publications; Philadelphia: J.B. Lippincott, 1990.

Zagelbaum G, Welch ME Jr, Doyle PR. *Basic Arterial Blood Gas Interpretation*. Little, Brown, Boston, 1988.

Index

Since one or more routine blood gas measurements (PaO_2, $PaCO_2$, etc.) or calculations (HCO_3^-, CaO_2, $P(A-a)O_2$, etc.) are mentioned on almost every page, these terms are indexed only on those pages that provide specific discussion or explanation. Also, because Quik-Course (Chapter 10) is a summary of the entire text, its pages are omitted from the index.

COMPUTER PROGRAMS

Over the years we have developed microcomputer programs for teaching pulmonary physiology and medicine. Two of these programs — Blood Gas Interpretation and Respiratory Failure Tutorial — are available by mail order for $20.00 U.S. (includes all postage and handling). Programs are available for IBM PC-compatible computers only (minimum requirement: 640 Kb RAM, DOS 2.1 or higher).

BLOOD GAS INTERPRETATION. Enter any of 25 blood gas, electrolyte and hemodynamic variables to obtain a computer-generated blood gas interpretation similar to those provided in Chapter 8. The program also calculates cardiopulmonary values such as systemic vascular resistance and % shunt. You can view the results on the screen or print them out.

RESPIRATORY FAILURE TUTORIAL. This multiple-choice, question and answer tutorial is designed to teach the basics of respiratory failure diagnosis and management. The program includes detailed explanations of both the correct and incorrect choices. The program also keeps score of your answers.

Both programs are included on one disk, either 3.5" or 5.25". To obtain the disk, please send a check or money order for $20.00 (U.S.) to the address below. Payment must accompany order. Credit cards cannot be accepted. Ohio residents, please add 7% sales tax ($1.40). Allow 3-4 weeks for delivery, longer for overseas delivery.

For both computer programs mail $20.00 (U.S.) by check or money order to:

> Mr. Brian Jeffreys
> 3842 Northwood Road
> University Heights, Ohio 44118

> Please indicate size of computer disk:
> ☐ 3.5"   ☐ 5.25"
